YOUR KEY TO A
HEALTHY HEART

*The Suppressed Record
of Vitamin E*

YOUR KEY TO A HEALTHY HEART

The Suppressed Record of Vitamin E

HERBERT BAILEY

CHILTON BOOKS

A DIVISION OF CHILTON COMPANY
Publishers
Philadelphia   New York

Second Printing, January 1965
Third Printing, April 1965
Fourth Printing, April 1966

DEDICATION

THIS BOOK is dedicated to those rare persons who honestly seek the truth in all of man's endeavors on this planet and will not allow egotism, personal gain, or seemingly insurmountable obstacles imposed by those in authority to deter them in the slightest from their quest.

He marched to the beat of a distant *drum*—Emerson.

Foreword

Man is an extraordinary creature which Nature has produced over a period of about a million years by slowly choosing from among the different kinds of human beings those whose physiology and mentality were best suited to the environment of the earth.

In the last several thousand years, man has used machines to reverse this process, changing his environment in the world to suit himself. This is a hazardous undertaking, because man's wisdom is too limited to foresee all the consequences of his acts. Some serious mistakes have been made, the insidious consequences of which were not easy to foresee. Today, of course, we live in the shadow of the ultimate disaster, which is the possible radioactive ruin of the earth.

One of the early, far reaching errors which man committed was described about 2,000 years ago by the Greek philosopher Plato. He called attention to ancient little temples still standing in the rather dry fields of Greece, and reminded his readers that in some earlier time these fields must have been fertile meadows because such temples were always built on the banks of running streams.

Thoughtless men over the years had cut down the mountain forests, the streams dried up, the land became arid, and a gifted people in a beautiful country suffered a disaster from which they have not yet recovered some twenty centuries later. China made a similar mistake, but her civilization survived on the great river deltas, and now she is making an immense effort to replant her mountain forests.

Almost a century ago, in 1870, humanity made another

major mistake which has caused a great deal of human misery and disease. This was the use of the high speed roller mill which removed the bran and germ, containing practically all the minerals and vitamins, from grain used in bread and other foods. The bran and germ were called the "offals," because nothing was known about vitamins, and the name persists to this day in the milling industry.

Only a few people appreciated that the "staff of life" had been emasculated. The new white flour made fluffy bread, and thorough advertising convinced the public that white was synonymous with good. Almost no insect could live on it, so the flour could be milled in a few places by powerful monopolies and shipped all over the world with almost no spoilage. Farmers found that the "offals" were wonderful for the health of livestock, which made white flour all the more profitable to the millers. The alteration of bread has now proceeded to the point where some seventy different chemicals are used in it, and practically all flour, white or whole, is devitalized by strong bleaching agents. Over twenty known vitamins or other beneficial substances are removed from flour; only about six or seven are replaced in today's so-called "enriched" bread. Significantly, Vitamin E is not among them. The entire process is a splendid commercial success. In the light of what we now know, it was also an unparalleled mistake in health which will probably take generations to overcome.

My own interest in Vitamin E was much increased about fifteen years ago, when I decided to make the diet of patients as simple and wholesome as possible. This decision was based, first, on the fact that in the case of animals, every farmer knows that his animals' diet is the most important factor in long range health. Second, I noticed that the quality of food many patients ate was inferior. B and E vitamins were deficient and sweet stuff was in excess. Third, orthodox medical treatment just did not produce long standing results in certain important common diseases. Finally, I found that I could often permanently relieve chronic colds by taking people off sweets, and often perma-

nently relieve chronic constipation and certain other gastro-
intestinal diseases by putting the patient on bread or cereal
made from freshly ground grains. Aged flour and cereal did not
have the same effect which suggests that vitamins, not merely
roughage, were doing the work.)

Results were even better if supplementary vitamin capsules
were added. I believe that years of relative vitamin neglect place
people, especially older people, in a sort of vitamin debt characterized by prematurely aged tissues and functions, a debt which
requires the intake of supplementary vitamins for a very considerable time.

The official medical propaganda against the use of Vitamin E
in heart disease discouraged me, along with most other doctors,
from using it specifically in that condition. But the evidence of
its favorable influence in cardiovascular and other diseases,
not only from the Dr. Shute brothers in Canada, but from
around the world, is now so extensive, and the theoretical basis
so sound, that a much more extensive clinical use of Vitamin E
should now be made in both prevention and treatment.

The author of this book has some severe criticisms of those
presently in control of official medical groups, such as the
American Medical Association, and governmental agencies,
such as the Food and Drug Administration, for their indifference
to Vitamin E. As the author has stated, on behalf of individual
doctors, it must be said that they are usually too busy extin-
guishing the acute fires of disease to have time to study or work
for major reforms in the field of health. Most have to rely solely
on AMA reports for their information. This should not be.
We are fortunate that a veteran medical reporter of Herbert
Bailey's skill and determination has provided a documented,
yet highly readable report for us on Vitamin E in this book.

With regard to the official position of the American Medical
Association, however, little can be said in the way of extenua-
tion. The AMA has plenty of time and facilities for scholarly
investigations, but we have learned that the leaders of this organization in the last twenty years have become much more

interested in expediency than in basic principles. Probably the chief and insidious reason for this is that the AMA has been much corrupted as a result of receiving in recent years over half its income from drug companies which advertise in its many journals. This serious conflict of interest tends to stifle broad and scholarly views on health, and to permeate all through the ramifications of AMA influence—in its journals, in industry, and in the governmental agencies which participate in the twenty-six billion dollars spent annually on health in this country.

We must look at the whole pattern in matters of health. Great industries have drifted into the production of things which at first seemed perfectly good. The degeneration and adulteration of processed foods and the creeping poisons in them, constitute changes in the human environment which have developed so gradually and on such a wide front that it is not easy to place the blame on any one commercial or professional group.

By the time humanity wakes up to its danger, the men involved are not only the victims of long habit, but also find that it is expensive or individually ruinous to change their ways. For self-preservation, they may mislead themselves and others and oppose reform as long as possible.

We are in need of a return to plain principles and simple remedies, in medicine and in our lives generally. We need to build less on sand and more on rock.

MILES H. ROBINSON, M.D.

Acknowledgments

A great number of persons have helped me in the preparation of this book, but I should like to render special credit to Mrs. Estelle Fine, whose remarkable talent for detailed questioning and editing contributed greatly to the publication of this book.

From the medical point of view, my particular appreciation goes to Dr. George Simmons, of New York City, who made cogent annotations which were duly appreciated and, for the most part, incorporated in the text. And I am deeply indebted to Dr. Miles Robinson, of Washington, D.C., and Potomac, Maryland, the author of the Foreword of this book, who has most generously aided the work by his suggestions and fearless presentation of the truth. Dr. Robinson, a specialist in internal medicine, is on the staff of the Washington Sanitarium and Hospital.

And, finally, to Neal Thorpe, my associate, whose assiduous labors in many libraries and investigations elsewhere and whose critical and creative editorial help were of inestimable benefit—my profound appreciation. Mr. Thorpe, being Vice-President of MAN's FRONTIERS, an organization which I founded a few years ago—"dedicated to explorations of the unknown and the dissemination of facts about hitherto generally suppressed subjects"—is truly dedicated to the service of his fellow man.

H. B.
Westport, Connecticut

Preface

Perhaps this preface should be termed a continuation of the dedication page, for that in reality is what it is. Those rare persons who seek the truth no matter where the pathways lead are in the heroic vanguard of the human race. They are the ones who take the bitter blows from Authority, the Status Quo, and the Establishment.

Today we are more than ever the victims of these Unholy Three because they have seized command in our times of virtually all the popular communications media—except books. The persons to whom I am dedicating this book know this full well. If this work succeeds in its purpose, I believe they can derive hope that their discoveries will have a better chance of receiving the fair treatment which they deserve. I believe that when enough persons take Vitamin E and recover from heart disease or prevent it, the majority will accept the facts and recognize the misrepresentations which have been an integral part of the Authority, the Status Quo, or the Establishment.

The problem of re-educating people is quite immense, but nevertheless I am convinced that it can be done. Let us start off with a very simple thesis: authorities, particularly those in the United States, are slow to accept basic changes.

How can those who are aware effect a change? Either by getting an influential leader to accept an effective yet unorthodox treatment or by so arousing the general public to the obvious truth that it will force the government to act. The latter of these alternatives is difficult because of the bureaucratic nature of governments. The former is even more difficult because unorthodox approaches have been so stigmatized and stamped out by the controlling medical bureaucracy that almost no one can believe that an unorthodox approach can have any validity. But we hope that this book will persuade enough people so that, in spite of the heavy odds, the truth will win out once again in the history of medicine.

Contents

YOUR KEY TO A
HEALTHY HEART

*The Suppressed Record
of Vitamin E*

1

My Personal Experience

My own heart attack occurred seven years ago on one of the finest days of my life. I had just returned from a leisurely, month-long trip, and feeling full of energy, I immediately set to wrestling huge logs up from the beach. I spent the whole day at this violent activity even though the logs were really too heavy for anyone in his right mind to tackle. But I was feeling the need for exercise which had long been frustrated, and so by the end of the day, working continuously, I had got the logs stacked neatly by our house. But when I came in for dinner, I collapsed.

I was suffering severe pains around the heart and I couldn't move. I seemed to be suffocating, but I could not breathe fast enough to overcome the awful sensation. I felt that I was going to die—altogether a most horrible, helpless, panicky feeling. Our excellent general practitioner and good friend was called in, and he immediately prescribed digitalis and nitroglycerine— plus absolute bed rest for at least three weeks. I was flabbergasted. I was working on an important book at the time and really needed every spare moment for hard labor. But he warned me that I had had a severe heart block and near failure due to congestion and that I required complete rest and no work at all. (A heart "block" means the pacemaker in the heart isn't transmitting properly; therefore, the necessary rhythm of the heart beat is disrupted.) I asked him about massive doses of Vitamin E which I had read about briefly somewhere, but he argued that he knew of no favorable literature on the subject for humans, just on rabbits and rats. We haggled a bit over the pros and cons of organized medicine, then he left me to my rest and digitalis.

While trying to follow his orders, I received the news via a courageous radio commentator and a courageous publisher that Vitamin E was in fact the best therapy for heart ailments of all types. I was informed that much literature on the subject was actually available; that, indeed, a book had been published by the pioneers of Vitamin E therapy, substantiating in great detail the proof of Vitamin E's efficacy in the treatment of heart and cardiovascular diseases.

Thus, my own heart attack was responsible for introducing me to the almost unknown remedy of Vitamin E for heart disease. I obtained the book, as well as some other literature, which was not an easy task. Also, the book was written for doctors. Its title was: *Alpha Tocopherol (Vitamin E) in Cardio-Vascular Disease*. It was compiled by Dr. Evan Shute and Dr. W. E. Shute of London, Ontario, Canada, but it included evidence from all over the civilized world. The senior author, Dr. Evan V. Shute, was then and still is a Fellow of the Royal College of Surgeons (Canadian), and each of the contributors in the clinical tests was a well-recognized M.D. There was one exception: N. M. Lambert, of Dublin, Ireland, who was then and is now a Fellow of the Royal College of Veterinary Surgeons. It was he who did the first work with Vitamin E on dogs and cats with heart disease, the astounding results of which we shall examine in due course.

Words cannot describe my reaction when I read the book. Although I was acutely aware of the adverse medical attitude toward any proposed cancer remedies by the medical "authorities," I was not prepared to admit that the suppression was also manifest in heart disease.

And yet there it was: Full and complete evidence on more than 10,000 heart disease victims which the non-profit Shute Foundation for Medical Research had treated in Canada. Many more thousands had been treated with beneficial results in other countries. (At this writing at least 60,000 persons throughout the world have been saved by Vitamin E therapy.) And this overwhelming evidence had been stifled, ignored, or, even worse, denied, in the medical press and, therefore, in the popular press as well. (These reports and references are available, however, in good medical libraries.)

I found out from Dr. Shute's book that I should probably take 600 international units of Vitamin E a day. I did.

On the third day of Vitamin E therapy, I felt a surge of energy, such a new awareness of physical well-being that I said to my wife, "I'll be damned if I'll stay in bed any longer." Nor did I. I got up and have never been confined to bed again because of heart trouble. And that is why seven years later, my digitalis and nitroglycerine tablets forgotten, I am able to take up the writing of this book. I am able today to work at my writing all through the night, to saw a few logs as the dawn comes up, and then to take a spin on my bicycle around the countryside without feeling any aftereffects except the exhilaration which comes from stimulating exercise. I know Vitamin E therapy is effective against almost all forms of cardiovascular ailments, unbelievable as it may seem. I want to pass on what I have learned so that others may benefit.

I know it will be difficult to convince everyone of the incredible value of Vitamin E—but I can try. In this book I shall refer to many of the actual cases which have been controlled or benefited by this vitamin. After reading it, go to your doctor, and if he says: "Don't pay any attention to this propaganda about Vitamin E; nothing has ever been published in this country which corroborates these wild, foreign claims" (an untrue statement; see Bibliography and Appendix), what are you going to do? My suggestion is that you follow exactly the same course I did back in 1957—take Vitamin E anyway. It's non-toxic.

In an experiment conducted at the State University of New York, College of Medicine, Brooklyn, New York, under the supervision of Dr. R. W. Hillman, a "normal" volunteer took two to four grams of Vitamin E daily for over three months.[1] (This dosage is two to four times the usual dosage for *treating*

---

[1] One gram is equivalent to 1,000 international units (I.U.), or 1,000 milligrams (mg.).

heart disease.) The results showed no lowering of exercise tolerance, and all other tests were normal—these included the electrocardiogram, ballistocardiogram, serum cholesterol, liver function, blood coagulation, and muscle biopsy—in short, most of the major tests known which would indicate even minor side-reactions or toxicity.

In addition, Dr. A. Del Giudice, of the National Institute of Public Health, Buenos Aires, has been giving two grams of Vitamin E daily for many years to retarded children—even Mongoloids. Not only has there been no evidence of toxic side effects, but Dr. Del Giudice has achieved some amazingly beneficent effects, both mental and physical.

All animal studies prove Vitamin E non-toxic per se, and all the official medical groups admit this fact. Finally, the authoritative *Taber's Cyclopedic Medical Dictionary* (1963, Ninth Edition) states that Vitamin E (Alpha-Tocopherol) is "non-toxic, even in large doses."

All this does *not* mean that you should gulp down a bottle full of Vitamin E capsules expecting the miracle cure in a day. The chances are such an imprudent act won't hurt you or help you. Any substance, including water, will kill you if you take enough of it. The wisdom of the ancient Greeks applies here, as in so many instances, "Everything in moderation, nothing to excess."

Now with this warning for those readers who are inclined toward excesses and who do not read beyond the first chapter, let us explore Vitamin E and what it does for animals as well as men. The probability is extremely high that Vitamin E can help you.

2

A Brief Review of the Scientific Evidence

Quite frankly, I wish I did not have to write this book. I had hoped that the medical profession, particularly in America, would have been impressed—even overwhelmed—by the monumental evidence presented in many hundreds of authenticated, scientific reports from all over the civilized world demonstrating that Vitamin E holds a major key to the control and prevention of most forms of heart disease, as well as many other diseases, as we shall demonstrate.

However, I have found that the vast majority of doctors in this country have a distorted concept of Vitamin E's efficacy. Why? Largely because the leaders of the organized medical fraternity have not seen fit to publish the favorable evidence in leading medical journals in the United States. Doctors who have been shown the evidence are amazed and cannot quite believe that such a dreadful suppression of the facts could happen here. They are even more amazed when they discover for themselves the hard, undeniable truth about Vitamin E's multi-faceted, heroic role in the body's metabolism, particularly in the heart muscle itself and in the circulatory system of every human being and every animal thus far studied. Throughout the past twenty years there have been hundreds of such studies; yet you will find that the majority of "cardiac" specialists have never read the available world literature on the subject. If they have read anything on Vitamin E, they consider it "controversial," and, therefore, not worthy of investigation. Unfortunately, in this country, the label "controversial" immediately brands any medical evidence as undesirable and discourages any further inquiries by individuals because they feel they must have complete professional approval.

Why the cardiac specialists and, therefore, the heart associations should be so unscientific concerning the most promising medical treatment for our most dreaded "killer" is a matter which we shall examine later. Our primary aim at this point is to present the evidence to both doctors and laymen so that everyone can see the extent of the misconceptions which have been perpetrated. I think I can prove to any scientist's satisfaction that the role of Vitamin E is no longer truly controversial in the scientific sense: that is, there exists an enormous amount of evidence supporting its value and effectiveness. What minimal amount of opposing evidence there is has usually resulted from inadequate dosages, incomplete testing, or use of synthetic Vitamin E[2] (which has now been shown to possess only approximately one-fifth the potency of the vitamin derived from natural sources). I will be footnoting some of the important statements in this summary chapter, and the reader will find adequate documentation of the scientific findings presented in the subsequent specialized chapters. These plus the extended bibliography will help those of scientific inclination to investigate the subject further. Let us now report on the scientific evidence that is available to all.

In 1959, the Federal Food and Drug Administration (FDA) begrudgingly admitted that Vitamin E is essential in human nutrition. Unfortunately, the FDA had been ignoring for twenty years the mass of evidence which had been accumulating from all over the world, including the United States. This government agency, however, rather than admit its mistake, covered it up by sending out a widely published press release stating that no one in this country need worry about a lack of Vitamin E—that anyone eating a "normal" diet obtains the minimum requirement. However, according to the researchers who were responsible for the FDA admitting the necessity of Vitamin E

[2] See Appendix C.

nutrition, this statement is extremely misleading. (Contrary to the FDA release, there are unassailable scientific studies[3] which demonstrate that from 5 to 7 per cent of adult Americans are deficient in Vitamin E.)

The FDA statement merely admits the value of the barest minimum one can exist on without showing obvious, unmistakable symptoms caused by an outright deficiency. What it failed to reveal was the pharmacodynamic action of Vitamin E on the body; by pharmacodynamic, I mean the action of the vitamin as used in the treatment and prevention of disease. The amounts involved are startlingly different.

Before we delve deeper into actual dosages used by the various researchers, we should examine the vitamin and its action in the body. Then we can understand Vitamin E's almost unlimited capacity for alleviating many of the ailments afflicting men.

What *is* Vitamin E and where is it found in nature?

Along with Vitamins A, D, and K, Vitamin E is oil-soluble and is found in the oils of wheat germ and many other plant seeds. It is also present to some degree in leafy vegetables and other plants. It is found in varying amounts in animal tissues (including man's), generally being concentrated in fatty tissues and in organs such as the heart and liver. Vitamin E is a vital component of the blood as well. Milk and eggs also contain the vitamin.

Vitamin E is composed of seven forms of what chemists term *tocopherols*. They are labeled *alpha, beta, gamma, delta, epsilon, eta,* and *zeta*—but *alpha* is the only form which has been shown to be very active in the animal or human body. Although the other tocopherols may someday be found to play a role in metabolism, as yet *alpha tocopherol* alone is synonymous with Vitamin E in the minds of most present-day re-

Note: Unless otherwise indicated, all footnotes refer to Bibliography.

[3] See P. L. Harris, *et al.;* also M. K. Horwitt, *et al., J. Am. Dietetic Assoc.*

searchers. By far the most significant results have been obtained in both animals and men, using only alpha tocopherol. In most substances from which tocopherols are derived, the alpha form comprises only 60 per cent of the total and sometimes much less; therefore, the dosage from a formula containing all the tocopherols must be nearly *doubled* in order to be therapeutically effective. This fact has been overlooked by many researchers as well as by the governmental agencies which maintain that everyone obtains enough Vitamin E in a "good, normal, healthy" diet and that, therefore, Vitamin E as a supplement is unnecessary. We shall demonstrate that not only are the official agencies ignoring the fact that alpha tocopherol is the only proven active factor in Vitamin E but that much more Vitamin E is necessary for even minimum daily requirements than is "officially" indicated. We shall show that an abundance of Vitamin E (alpha tocopherol) can and does prevent, as well as control, many ailments known to man, and to beast, both feral and domesticated.

Henceforth, when we use the term Vitamin E, we are referring to alpha tocopherol, not to the other inactive forms of the vitamin.

It has been established by many researchers (and accepted by all researchers) that Vitamin E is an "anti-oxidant" and an oxygen-conservator. These properties signify that Vitamin E possesses the ability to improve the cell's function and prolong its life. As an anti-oxidant, Vitamin E delays the oxidative process which turns cells "rancid," and it prevents oxygen from combining with other substances to form the deadly hydrogen peroxide which hastens the death of a cell. This fact has been proven on human beings, on animals, and on tissues which have been removed from recently-killed animals.

When the facts are established on living humans and animals, the study is called an experiment *in vivo*. *In vitro* is the term used when the experiment is performed *outside* the living organism, as for instance when the heart of a frog is removed from the animal's body to determine how much longer the heart will beat when it is bathed in a solution containing Vitamin E as compared with the time it will continue to beat when bathed in a saline solution. Researchers have found that the frog's heart is so strengthened by Vitamin E that the heart beat is prolonged by nearly 50 per cent. Other muscle tissues of the frog and other animals as well are equally strengthened by addition of Vitamin E.

Human red blood cells offer another example of *in vitro* work. Dr. M. K. Horwitt at Elgin State Hospital in Elgin, Illinois, found that human red blood cells when adequately supplied with Vitamin E do not lose their hemoglobin (an oxygen-carrying material) nearly as fast as cells deficient in Vitamin E.[4] This means that red blood cells maintain their integrity (and, therefore, their lives) much longer than cells which are not amply supplied with Vitamin E. These facts are of utmost significance, as we shall see. (Parenthetically, it has been suggested that Vitamin E be used in the preservation of blood now stored in blood banks since the present "shelf-life" of such stored whole blood is relatively short.[5] It has also been found that meats of animals fed Vitamin E supplements will "keep" much longer than ordinary meats.)

A natural anti-oxidant and oxygen-conservator such as Vitamin E affords the body many advantages. First, when richly supplied with Vitamin E, the cells of the body are able to perform more efficiently—not demanding as much oxygen for metabolic processes, thereby freeing more oxygen for those cells and organs needing it. An ailing heart, for instance, not demanding as much oxygen as before—that is, before the therapeutic dose of Vitamin E—does not have to pump as hard to convey blood to the cells. Its work is considerably lessened, consequently easing the strain—an extremely important factor in heart ailments. Also, the heart muscle itself is more richly nourished with oxygen through its main source of blood supply, the coronary arteries. These two factors—less work and more

---

[4] M. K. Horwitt, *et al.*, *Federation Proc.*
[5] See Bibliography: Meyer-Wegener and Luzak.

oxygen—partially explain why the vitamin has a direct, beneficial, seemingly miraculous, effect on flagging hearts, and on
normal hearts as well. Researchers have stated that Vitamin E
therapy is equivalent to being placed in an oxygen tent—without
the inconvenience, of course.

But equally as important as its oxygen-hoarding properties
is the fact that Vitamin E "guides" oxygen in proper functions.
When cells have a scarcity of Vitamin E, they tend to release
their oxygen, which then combines with the cellular wastes to
form poisons deadly to the cells—hydrogen peroxide among
others—which rapidly destroy red blood cells as well as the
enzyme *catalase* which is vital to aeration of the cells.

Vitamin E is also a vasodilator: it opens arteries (particularly those all-important smallest ones, the arterioles) so that
more blood can flow through the circulatory system. This is of
particular significance to victims of circulatory disorders such as
arteriosclerosis and *atherosclerosis*. (*Arteriosclerosis* is the general term employed to encompass almost all disorders of the
arterial and venous system which are considered to be due to
"aging." More specifically, the term refers to "hardening" and
"thickening" of the arteries, accompanied by loss of elasticity in
the blood vessels. *Atherosclerosis* is characterized by "clogging"
of the arteries with fatty deposits on the walls. Often these deposits break away in "chunks" through the action of the heart,
which has an increasingly difficult job of forcing blood through
increasingly narrowing arteries. If such a piece of material [a
"clot" or "thrombus"] makes its way to the heart and/or blocks
the flow of blood to the heart, then we have one of the most
common forms of the dread "coronary thrombosis.")

The foregoing attributes of Vitamin E help to explain why
rats, guinea pigs, race horses, and humans develop much more
endurance than the "normal" when given large amounts of
Vitamin E in the diet. For instance, Vitamin E-treated rats
can swim nearly twice as long as non-treated animals and can
withstand high altitudes which quickly kill their own litter
mates. Humans tested on a "treadmill" and elsewhere show

the same increased endurance when their diets are supplemented heavily with Vitamin E.

Still another faculty of Vitamin E is its anti-coagulant (anti-blood-clotting) power. Moreover, this anti-coagulant quality of the vitamin does not produce harmful side-effects as do the drugs heparin and dicumarol, which are now in common use in an attempt to treat and prevent the formation of clots—the clots (thrombi) being the leading cause of "coronaries" and "strokes," whether they be due to the formation of blood clots or to "flaking" away of the fatty deposits. The latter drugs must be used with extreme caution, for they tend to produce hemorrhages. There is great debate raging in the medical world as to whether these drugs should be used *at all,* as their action of artificially creating *hemophilia* (bleeding which is extremely difficult to control) seems to outweigh their merit as anti-coagulants. (See Appendix A, pages 150–151.)

With Vitamin E, however, such is not the case no matter how massive the dosage employed. Further, Vitamin E has shown some propensity to *dissolve* clots. Although Vitamin E is also a dependable, efficient anti-coagulant, its action stops when its anti-blood-clotting ability is no longer needed; indeed, it even hastens wound healing and tends to prevent scars and occasionally even dissolves scar tissue. (See Chapter 6.)

Still another recognized property of the amazing Vitamin E is its ability to maintain normal permeability of cellular membranes, notably the capillaries. You will recall that capillaries are the tiny blood vessels which supply nourishment to individual cells. If the capillary walls become too impermeable, their function of feeding the cells is impaired; on the other hand, if the walls become too permeable, they leak out their precious cargo into the extra-cellular spaces where it does not belong, and, thus, the cells are deprived of nutrition. So we see that a constant supply of the proper substances is needed to sustain the tricky equilibrium maintained between the capillaries and the cells. Along with other substances such as Vitamin C and the bioflavonoids, Vitamin E maintains the normal integrity of these walls, preventing them from becoming too permeable or impermeable, or from "breaking."

Thus we see Vitamin E's essential role—or multiple roles —at the most vital cellular level. We can begin to understand why the vitamin in therapeutic quantities should be effective in many ailments. Admittedly, there is very little going on in this wondrously wrought mind-body-brain we call a human being that would not be affected by oxygen-conserving, clot-dissolving, wound-healing, and blood-vessel normalizing.

In fact, Vitamin E is so effective against so many diseases that it seems almost incredible—were it not for the knowledge we have acquired about its basic, specific and non-specific actions. It is, indeed, somewhat of a panacea, in the best sense of the word. Yet it is not a "cure-all." It will not keep you from dying, but it will prevent or control many diseases now troubling man, and, based on the experience of thousands who have been taking Vitamin E for years, it will make life worth living for a longer period.

The list of diseases which Vitamin E has been reported to improve and/or control is seemingly endless. We shall merely mention several of them, without, at this point, delving into theoretical considerations or analyzing the experiments. (See Chapter 6 for more details.)

Many researchers have recorded that diabetes is often controlled or semi-controlled by Vitamin E. Many patients have been able to dispense with insulin entirely while others have had its use drastically reduced. If this fact were to become more widely known, it would very likely result in the alleviation of much of the suffering which millions of persons now have to endure because of this misunderstood, yet common, disease.

Vitamin E has been demonstrated to be of considerable value in treating the symptoms of menopause—the "change of life" which countless women find almost unbearable. (See Bibliography, *Journal American Medical Association*.) It has been dubbed "nature's own tranquilizer," by various gynecologists, who have found that heavy doses of Vitamin E somewhat approximate the effects of estrogen—the female hormone—in relieving "hot flashes," nervousness, depression, anxiety, and irritability without the adverse side effects of the hormone.

Vitamin E has also been used in preventing habitual abortions,[6] as well as the tragedy of congenitally deformed babies. Several series of experiments have shown that childless couples when given massive treatments of Vitamin E (and this means both the man and the woman) can very often have children, when nothing else was effective.[7]

Eye disorders in children[8] (near-sightedness, crossed eyes), along with mental retardation, have been reported corrected or alleviated with extremely large doses of Vitamin E (up to 3,000 international units a day for years).

It has been responsible for preventing and curing cirrhosis and other disorders of the liver in so many laboratory animals of all types that the implication for man cannot be ignored.[9] Several studies on man will be reviewed in Chapter 6.

Vitamin E has been found to be of marked value in the treatment of such obscure and remote diseases as leprosy[10] (Hansen's disease); lupus erythematosus[11] (a tuberculosis skin disease which is characterized by an intractable rash); and in the prevention of sickness due to X-ray therapy.

Vitamin E has been shown to have a close relationship to muscular dystrophy,[12] indications being that, in muscular dystrophy, the body cannot assimilate the vitamin properly. There is some reason to believe that, once a key to the proper assimilation of Vitamin E is found for the unfortunate victims of muscular dystrophy, they will be cured much as victims of the

---

[6] See Sutton; Boyer.

[7] Da Rugna; Horne; Brown, *et al.*

[8] Desusclade; Sbordone; Vannas and Orma.

[9] Bechman; Stormont, *et al.;* Hadnagy, *et al.;* Rodnan, *et al.*

[10] De Campos Magalhaes and Figueiredo Barbosa; Sarmento; Bergel; Floch and Horth; Mason and Bergel.

[11] Its use in various skin diseases: Walther; Nikolowski; Frey; Grubb; Kimmig.

[12] Nielsen and Marvin; Gros and Kirnberger; Shcherbakova.

once-fatal pernicious anemia are now cured by injections of Vitamin B-12 and the mysterious "intrinsic factor," which is derived from gut tissue.

At least one study (from Tehran, Iran, by H. Davidian) has shown that Vitamin E is valuable in the withdrawal from drug addiction.

There is evidence that Vitamin E tends to normalize blood pressure in some persons, bringing the pressure up if it is too low, and down if it is too high. (See Chapter 8.)

There is also some evidence that Vitamin E can prevent or at least slow down the formation of so-called "old age" deposits in the cells and tissues—the "ceroid" pigmentation and "granular" formations. As an animal (or human) grows older, the cells, organs, and tissues become increasingly permeated with inactive substances which are no doubt due to the gradual diminution of the metabolic processes. In countless laboratory tests, Vitamin E has shown its ability to reverse or slow down this aging process.[13] Some researchers hold that these inert, inactive substances which gradually fill space in the cell—which should be occupied by vital, active, and working substances—are the actual primary cause of death. These inert, useless "cell fillers" slowly choke off the useful, efficient materials which are occupied in the process of keeping us alive and healthy. Therefore, if Vitamin E can manage to halt or, at least, delay this detrimental aging process, it follows that man may live to his true (mammalian) span of about 150 years in full vigor instead of slowly creeping to his grave—as Shakespeare puts it so aptly: "sans teeth, sans eyes, sans everything." A study of all mammals on the earth from rats to elephants shows that mammals—barring accidents—live about six times their maturation rate. For instance, a dog, which is fully matured in two years, usually lives about twelve years; thus man, maturing at twenty-five, should live to be 150.

There are excellent scientific indications that Vitamin E can be the most potent single factor in warding off old age—pro-

[13] Aslan; Morgan.

vided one obtains enough and can utilize it efficiently. Individuals vary so much in their demand for any nutritive substance that an individual (or a doctor) has to proceed by trial or by subjective and/or objective results in order to determine how much of any substance is needed. We have not yet achieved the robot stage whereby a standard squirt of Vitamin E (or other necessary material) will suffice to keep all the machines in good working order. It has been ascertained that the human utilizes only about 20 to 30 per cent of the Vitamin E he ingests. Therefore, some persons have to take more than others for the vitamin to be effective.

These are some of the major functions scientists *know* about Vitamin E. There are many other functions, some of which, at present, they do not know; yet because the vitamin does produce observable reactions in animals and humans, researchers can make educated guesses.

Now let us explore a short history of the vitamin and try to ascertain why there has been such a time lag between its actual discovery and its widespread clinical acceptance and use.

3

Vitamin E's Challenging History

Vitamin E was discovered in 1922 by researchers H. M. Evans and K. S. Bishop. Unfortunately for human beings, but perhaps fortunately for science in the long run, these researchers picked the rat to prove the existence of the then unnamed substance. Had they chosen other animals, the results of Vitamin E deprivation would not have been the same as they were in the rat. The goat, for instance, apparently manufactures its own Vitamin E (just as the dog manufactures its own Vitamin C); however, in all other animals tested (sixteen thus far) deprivation of Vitamin E caused serious disorders—and finally death.

The original researchers chose the laboratory rat because its nutritional needs are somewhat close to man's. The rat is, like man, an omnivore, *i.e.,* it eats almost anything including meat, vegetables, and grains. The rat is even closer to man, nutritionally speaking, than most other species, including our "closest relatives," the apes, which eat vegetables and fruits primarily. The apes will not eat meat; neither will the horse or elephant, which may partially explain why these animals in the natural state have to spend practically all their waking time eating or looking for food. They have to supply their need for protein by eating large quantities of vegetation, rather than obtaining it in its concentrated form, which is meat, or animal products.

Vitamin E is absolutely essential for the rat in order to achieve reproduction. Certain other adult animals, such as chickens,[14] lambs, and cows, if deprived of Vitamin E, *may*

[14] Grabowsky.

16

reproduce, but their *offspring* never get a chance to reproduce. The reason? Vitamin E-starved chicks die of "crazy chick disease" (encephalomalacia), a disorder of the brain; lambs deprived of Vitamin E die of "stiff-lamb disease," within days or weeks; minks and mink kits die of "yellow fat" disease. Reproduction is thus eliminated in the second generation because these animals die before they can reproduce. If the rat is deprived of Vitamin E, it either cannot reproduce or else the foetus is "resorbed" by the mother and there is no birth at all.

This was a seemingly significant discovery at the time. It still is significant in the light of later research. However, the implication for the human being concerning reproduction was not long in being deduced. Vitamin E became known as the "fertility" vitamin. Then rapidly, because of the peculiar way that our society is constituted, Vitamin E achieved the medical status of being ranked along with Voronoff's "monkey glands" as a sexual rejuvenator. It is difficult to believe, in view of the thousands of reports published since then concerning its diverse roles in metabolism, that there are still some medical "authorities" who think of Vitamin E *only* as a "fertility" substance. It does happen that some humans, both man and woman, are affected beneficially by Vitamin E in the reproductive process,[15] but that is a relatively minor factor—almost a side effect—of the vitamin when compared with its other capacities.

At first, Vitamin E was also thought to be synonymous with wheat germ oil, but although wheat germ oil does contain some Vitamin E, the amount is usually not enough for therapeutic or even preventive dosages for the major degenerative diseases. But this fact was to be learned much later after many experiments and many scientific arguments. (Wheat germ oil, however, has additional stamina-building qualities other than that contained in Vitamin E and should be taken in conjunction with Vitamin E.)

Thus, there were double anathemas cast upon Vitamin E;

[15] See Chapter 6.

namely, (1) it was a "sexual" vitamin and, therefore, could not be tolerated in an ostensibly Puritanical society where sex was a dirty word; and (2) the early researchers did not have Vitamin E in sufficient quantities (they were using wheat germ oil). These early experiments were also confined to rats and rabbits for the most part, which hampered progress even more. And no one knew then that the wheat germ oil being used was probably turning rancid and, therefore, almost useless since rancidity not only destroys Vitamin E but has a most significant adverse effect on cellular metabolism.

However, to add an even more devastating road block in the path of the researchers, in 1937 Vitamin E was finally synthesized as a chemical laboratory product and more researchers began to use it, but no one was to know until 1962 that the synthetic product would be proved by the strictest tests to be only one-fifth as powerful as the product derived from natural sources. Meanwhile, many researchers were using the synthetic product and claiming little results. (See Appendix C.)

Most of the early workers were trying to establish Vitamin E's efficacy, or lack of it, in various types of animals and in the human—purely on its relationship to fertility—without having enough (as we know now) of the vitamin to make a valid test even on the reproductive basis. Yet these tests of twenty to thirty years ago are the ones now accepted and quoted by the medical authorities to prove that Vitamin E is worthless for the human body as a therapeutic agent *of any kind*.

There were a few pioneers during this period who used Vitamin E for various ailments and who obtained good results, but, regrettably, these findings were never followed up. Therefore, Vitamin E encountered a long dry spell between 1922 and 1945, when Dr. Evan V. Shute of London, Ontario, Canada, began seriously to investigate Vitamin E. In the book, *Alpha Tocopherol* [Vitamin E] *in Cardiovascular Disease* (1954), he describes how he arrived on the scene by a "series of lucky accidents." He had been intrigued by Vitamin E some years before (1936) but had "ignored the clues."

Now, Dr. Shute, a Fellow of the Royal College of Surgeons (Canada) is one of Canada's most respected physicians. He is an obstetrician and gynecologist, but his interests in medicine are far-ranging. His brother, Wilfrid, also a physician, leans more toward cardiovascular diseases.

Evan, as a child in Canada, qualified at a very early age for the rank of genius. He entered high school at the age of nine, a feat never surpassed in Canada. He sailed through high school, obtaining the highest standing in Essex County, Ontario, and then won a scholarship to the University of Toronto at the age of 14—another record never before achieved in Canada. He received his Bachelor of Arts degree in 1924 and three years later, his medical degree.

In 1933, Dr. Shute was made a Diplomate of the American Board of Obstetrics and Gynecology, which is quite an honor for a young physician. However, an even greater accolade was to follow two years later: he was selected as a Fellow of the Royal College of Surgeons (Canadian). Other honors followed in rapid succession, which we will not enumerate here due to lack of space, but we must mention that he has authored over 120 medical papers and has lectured at international medical meetings in London, New York, Naples, Venice, and Amsterdam. He is also listed in Canada's *Who's Who,* the *Directory of Medical Specialists, American Men of Science,* and *American Men of Medicine.*

We felt it necessary to acquaint the reader with Dr. Shute's accomplishments and recognitions in the field of orthodox medicine so that no one could possibly question his medical background. Now we will return to the history of his discovery.

Together, the brothers Shute had begun treatment of cardiovascular diseases with Vitamin E as early as 1936–37 but, as they term these studies now, they were "abortive." Preparations of the substance were poor and lack of facilities curtailed their research. Nevertheless the results obtained were so suggestive that they never forgot them.

In 1945, due to a brilliant type of research which Dr. Evan

Shute proposed to a doctoral candidate, Floyd Skelton, the intriguing question of Vitamin E's efficacy in the matter of blood coagulation arose. Purpura (a bad breakage of the smaller blood vessels) was induced in dogs—the animals chosen for the experiment—and then relieved by large doses of Vitamin E. Skelton's (now Dr.) research proved so fascinating that Dr. Shute resolved to try Vitamin E on a human patient. The patient they selected was in the last stages of purpura. His doctors were considering removing his spleen in the hope that somehow the condition could be helped.

Now, removal of the spleen is a most serious operation—for the patient, that is—since the spleen is foremost among those organs and tissues which comprise the body's natural line of defense against infections and diseases of all types. This natural defense mechanism is termed the *reticulo-endothelial system* (R.E.S.). Among the R.E.S.'s many activities is the manufacture of antibodies and white corpuscles.

An operation, however, was not actually possible since the patient had severe heart failure. You cannot remove a man's spleen when he is suffering desperately from heart disease. Therefore, researcher Skelton and Dr. Shute, calculating on the basis of the dosage used to cure the dogs of purpura, administered 200 I.U. of Vitamin E a day to their despairing patient. This dosage was much higher than had ever been used before in treating human beings. Today we know this dosage is extremely low; it helps to explain why some researchers could not obtain uniform or even satisfactory results.

Even so, the patient's heart trouble quickly disappeared—*before* his purpura, though that, too, yielded under the onslaught of the then mysterious substance called Vitamin E.

You can imagine Dr. Shute's thoughts at the miracle accomplished by the administration of a *mere* vitamin, the dosage of which would appear as an infinitesimal speck in the palm of a man's hand. Reacting as a true scientist, he immediately looked about for more patients—only those with heart disease this time—on whom he could again test Vitamin E.

He did not have far to look. His erstwhile barber was now dying from recurrent coronary thrombosis (the disease which kills more than half the men over 45). The barber was in the last stages of heart failure, complicated by a type of angina which was extremely painful and which no anodyne could relieve. Now anyone who has suffered angina knows it is one of the most "painful pains" known to man and also one of the most terrifying. When you know it is your heart which is sending out this most urgent call for relief, it is a slightly different matter from suffering from any other pain. You know, for instance, that the almost unendurable pain experienced in the aftermath of a torn-off leg or even that of a migraine headache will eventually disappear and that your life will be saved if you are in competent medical hands. But, in this case, you know that if your heart stops functioning, *you* stop functioning also.

There are millions of persons who are now enduring exactly the same type of pain from the same type of disease which Dr. Shute's barber was suffering in 1945. Very likely they could have been helped if Dr. Shute's findings had become common knowledge in that year and in the succeeding years. Fortunately for Dr. Shute's dying barber, after being treated with Vitamin E for three weeks, *he was playing the drums in one of the local theaters*. We may assume that he had returned to his regular profession of cutting hair as well, although this information is not vouchsafed to us by Dr. Shute in his book.

Next, the Shute brothers treated their mother with Vitamin E. She was suffering from severe *angina pectoris*. Again the vitamin worked; their mother's gripping pains ceased, and she was able to resume her normal activities.

Encouraged by these results (and who wouldn't be?), the Shute brothers, with the assistance of Dr. Arthur Vogelsang, a general practitioner and former student of Dr. Evan Shute, began a series of treatments on persons suffering from cardiovascular diseases.

Their results were as phenomenal as those previously described. At the time of compiling their monumental work in

1954, Drs. Shute, *et al.,* had treated more than 10,000 heart patients—with fantastic, scarcely-credible results (now over 20,000). Overnight the picture of gloom which had pervaded the whole area of heart disease was changed into the bright, glowing colors of optimism. At least that is what the Shutes thought. And that is, of course, what should have occurred.

But the Shutes had to learn the hard way. One would have expected that the medical profession and the medical journals would have seized upon this radical discovery when it was backed up by the most careful type of scientific evidence. This evidence included, naturally, the living, now normal patients who had been doomed to die. The patients possessed undeniable records of their illness as well as physical proof of their return to healthy living. Almost none of the diagnoses of heart disease were made initially by the Shutes—these were patients given up as "hopeless" by cardiac specialists.

The Shutes expected that the medical journal to which they sent their report would be proud to be the *first* medical journal to break the news to doctors—and therefore the world—that finally a *real key to heart disease* had been found with indisputable proof. To their amazement the Shutes' report was rejected. The doctors thought there must be some mistake. However, the second medical journal refused to publish also, as did the third. As Dr. Evan Shute puts it in his book in a classic masterpiece of understatement: "To give some slight indication of our problem, we once had resigned ourselves to being unable to publish our work in any medical journal. We sought unsuccessfully to register our manuscripts with the National Research Council of Canada, planning then to retire from this field of endeavor."

However, "The Council felt unable to assist us in this way, so we *perforce* continued our studies." (The italics are mine.) The Shutes were forced to continue their research with Vitamin E because they could not abandon their search for the truth in spite of official scepticism and opposition. They eventually founded the non-profit Shute Foundation for Medical Research and have since 1954 treated successfully many thousands of heart disease sufferers. They have collected reports from all over the world, attesting to the value of Vitamin E not only in heart disease but in many other ailments afflicting human beings.

As Dr. Shute relates it in his book, heart specialists (cardiologists) condemned his findings at first sight without ever reading the evidence. Similar experiences have occurred to other scientists. Witness Dr. Émil Grubbé's long fight to gain acceptance for X-ray therapy which he discovered in 1896, only a few weeks after Roentgen made his monumental discovery of the mysterious, invisible rays. Although Grubbé had demonstrated clearly on the first patient that X-rays were capable of shrinking cancer and relieving pain, the findings were bitterly attacked by the orthodox groups, particularly the surgeons.

Almost everyone who issues medical information emanating from orthodox sources or writes directly from their press handouts conveniently ignores the scandalous fact that X-ray was not recognized as an agent for treating cancer by the American College of Surgeons until 1937! And that Dr. Grubbé, the discoverer of X-ray therapy (for cancer and other diseases) *still* was not recognized as late as 1951! A former medical pupil of Dr. Grubbé's (Dr. George Park, a researcher and also a practicing physician in Chicago) informed me in the early part of 1951 of this shameful neglect on the part of the medical profession.

I investigated this and found the startling tale to be, indeed, true; Dr. Grubbé, then living in obscurity and suffering from X-ray burns incurred before anyone knew that the mysterious, invisible rays could damage human flesh, produced all the scientific evidence, all the documentation necessary to prove that he was the first man on our planet to apply Roentgen's discovery to medical healing. (Actually, Grubbé had been experimenting with X-rays *before* Roentgen announced his finding; Grubbé had been badly burned by X-rays previously in his experiments with Crookes' tubes, which generated radiation though no one knew what radiation was at that time.)

I wrote the tragic story of Grubbé for *Pageant* magazine (August, 1951). It was picked up by the wire services; radio and TV appearances followed. And *this* was how Dr. Grubbé was finally recognized by the orthodox medical groups. After the "forced" recognition, the old doctor was then fêted, awarded medals, and, before he died, became acknowledged as "one of our greatest medical pioneers."

I think it is apropos of our story of Vitamin E to relate this modern saga of neglect and eventual recognition by the medical "authorities." The authorities had fought and then ignored Dr. Grubbé so long that he had been, indeed, forgotten.

When I asked Dr. Grubbé what he thought was the reason for the authorities' fighting the X-ray for so long, he replied bluntly: "The surgeons. They controlled medicine, and they regarded the X-ray as a threat to surgery. At that time surgery was the only approved method of treating cancer. They meant to keep it the *only* approved method by ignoring or rejecting any new methods or ideas. This is why I was called a 'quack' and nearly ejected from hospitals where I had practiced for years."

By the time the American College of Surgeons was finally forced to admit that radiation therapy did not constitute a threat to surgery—indeed was most often a necessary part of the orthodox treatment of cancer—it was much too embarrassing for their leaders to recognize a man who had been persecuted by them for forty-one years. It was much more convenient to ignore him altogether in the hope that no one would ever drag *that* skeleton out of their medical closet.

It is ironic that the radiologists who are now under the protective aegis of the AMA, *et al.,* have no concept of their indebtedness to a courageous pioneer who made their good living possible and that these same doctors are now in the forefront of those who are fighting any other unorthodox approach to the treatment of cancer.

Another classic example of such authoritative thinking occurred in 1934. This was related to me by Dr. Frederic Gibbs of the University of Illinois College of Medicine. Dr. Gibbs is today recognized as being the pioneer who introduced the electroencephalograph (EEG) in this country. (The EEG was developed by Dr. Hans Berger of Austria.) Now, of course, the EEG is used routinely in the mapping of the brain, and it has led, and is leading, us to many valuable clues in the diagnosis and treatment of several diseases, such as brain tumor, epilepsy, and other disorders. Also, the EEG is considered one of man's most valuable tools in discovering the brain's functions under many circumstances, such as sleeping, dreaming, waking, hypnosis, insanity—to mention a few. Dr. Gibbs exhibited his then esoteric machine at the annual American Medical Association meeting in 1934.

Need we spell out what happened at that fateful meeting? Again, the medical profession failed to recognize the value of a new discovery. It was declared a "fake" by a doctor, who wildly flailed his arms and went into all sorts of emotional routines. Of course, we now know the value of the EEG, but it was left to researchers in England, Europe, and a few in the United States (including Gibbs) to begin the long arduous task of developing a promising science. The weight of their findings finally forced the advocates of the status quo in medicine to accept the EEG. (An interesting footnote to the now accepted reputation of Dr. Gibbs was his being called as an expert witness in the use of the EEG to testify in the trial of Jack Ruby, the slayer of Lee Oswald, the alleged assassin of the late President Kennedy. Gibbs testified that Ruby was suffering from an extremely rare—but undeniable—form of epilepsy: psychomotor.)

These few, yet meaningful examples of how the progress of modern medicine has been impeded will prepare the reader for what follows in the case of Vitamin E. What happened to Dr. Shute after publication of his book in 1954? Remember the heart disease cases treated by the Shutes *alone* by that time totaled 10,000. Other eminent researchers had treated thousands more. Almost all had attested to the marvelous effect of

Vitamin E. Dr. Shute thought the final victory of Vitamin E would be secured by publication of such overwhelming evidence.

He wrote: "Its [Vitamin E's] place as an essential item in normal cardiovascular physiology seems to have been firmly established . . . however we can testify that this has been an exhilarating if exhausting chase. And we know how a fox feels." As time proved, Dr. Shute was underestimating the hunters. They would not withdraw from the chase in spite of the publication of an enormous amount of favorable scientific evidence. He was to learn that no matter how much evidence he and his fellow researchers would amass during the next decade, the organized groups would ignore and deprecate all such evidence. Further, he would learn to his sorrow that mere deprecation and adverse aspersions would not be all he (and other workers) would suffer.

It must have come as a great shock to the Drs. Shute to learn that doctors in their own city of London, Ontario, who had witnessed firsthand the amazing results of Vitamin E and who were indeed using it *themselves,* were not prescribing it for their patients! And most of those "courageous" few who did prescribe it for their patients made their prescriptions valid only in another city because they did not wish to be known as a doctor who prescribes Vitamin E! To the uninitiated, this may seem incredible; yet the record stands and is there for all to see. This amazing fact—though somewhat disillusioning to followers of TV's hero doctors—was printed in *Maclean's Magazine,* one of Canada's foremost popular publications. It was later recounted in *Prevention* magazine in order that American readers might obtain some of the sordid, yet factual and realistic, circumstances surrounding today's practice of medicine. (See Appendix B for full details.)

The article must have shocked the American public, which is used to hearing the authorities proclaiming that the conquest of heart disease is just around the corner but that there are as yet no known remedies for heart disease or circulatory disease except those now in common use. Readers of popular magazines and viewers of television programs have been told the same story over and over again. All these media ignored the mountains of facts about Vitamin E which have been accumulating during the past twenty years.

A slight break in this wall of resistance occurred in the fall of 1959 when the United States Food and Drug Administration was forced to recognize that Vitamin E was just as essential to the welfare of the human body as vitamins A, D, the B-complex, and several other vitamins are acknowledged to be. For twenty odd years, this agency had been ignoring the evidence, following the practice of the orthodox medical groups. Far from having any favorable effects on heart disease, such as those reported by the Drs. Shute and hundreds of other researchers, the vitamin was not even deemed necessary for normal metabolism in the human being. In fact, prior to the 1959 ruling, the FDA would seize any Vitamin E product which carried a claim that it *was* essential in human nutrition.

However, as we have stated previously, when researchers, such as Dr. M. K. Horwitt at the Elgin State Hospital in Elgin, Illinois, proved conclusively that a deficiency of Vitamin E in the blood of the human being produces the destruction of red blood cells, the FDA statement was released. (There *are* courageous researchers in this country who pursue their experiments in spite of official opinion, and these are the ones we have to thank for our knowledge of many new medical developments.)

The release was, in effect, a counter-attack on those researchers who had demonstrated that Vitamin E was essential in human nutrition, for it stated that while Vitamin E had been officially declared as necessary in human nutrition, there was absolutely no need for anyone to be concerned about it since everyone in America received an ample supply of Vitamin E in his daily diet. In fact, judging from the stories in the press, one received the impression that Vitamin E was of no real importance at all. The FDA press release went even further, disparaging those researchers who maintained that massive doses of Vitamin E would benefit the body at all. The solid records of Shute and many other researchers in every civilized country in the world were dismissed as "wild claims."

Of course, Dr. Shute was dismayed by the sheer effrontery of any official agency which could blithely dismiss all the positive evidence for Vitamin E and, indeed, use the occasion of its admission to the official list of "necessary" vitamins as a springboard for a vicious attack against it. The top FDA officials are also quick to attach the label "quack" or "food faddist" to anyone who maintains that extra supplements of vitamins should be included in the diet. Yet the fallacy in this line of attack is adequately revealed by the numerous clinical studies reported in the medical journals. The frequency of these reports is only exceeded by the almost countless number of advertisements for vitamin supplements in these same medical journals. These reports and ads, of course, are rarely seen by the public.

It seems that vitamin supplements are excellent, indeed, if prescribed by a physician, but highly unnecessary if the individual takes them on his own.

In the case of Vitamin E, here is a letter from Dr. Shute sent to the Better Business Bureau concerning the FDA release and the subsequent BBB Service Bulletin based upon the release:

January 5, 1960

NATIONAL BETTER BUSINESS BUREAU, INC.
CHRYSLER BUILDING
NEW YORK 17, N.Y.
Dear Sirs:

I have just seen the little Service Bulletin of November 4th last, which deals with "Wild Claims for Vitamin E."

As so many of these so-called "wild claims" have emanated from me in the last 15 years, it is probably right that I should make some comment on your little item. The first thing that I should point out to you, perhaps, is that these "wild claims" have received so much credence now, that the writer has discussed them by invitation at international meetings in many countries in the last few years, including the Third World Congress on Vitamin E at Venice in 1955, the Third International Congress on Fertility and Sterility in Naples in 1956, as well as the Second of these Congresses held in New York in 1953, the World Congress on Angiology at San Remo in 1958, and the World Congress on Fertility and Sterility in Amsterdam in 1959. On January 12th next I am to give a lecture by invitation on "The Uses of Vitamin E in Obstetrics and Vascular Disease" at the Pan-American Fertility Congress in Miami Beach. There also have been many publications on this topic in English-speaking medical journals throughout the world. You can see, therefore, that perhaps these [claims] are not quite so "wild" as the FDA would suggest.

Now let me give some information on the background of some other remarks in your Service Bulletin. You begin by quoting the hoary old chestnut that "the daily diet provides more than adequate amounts of Vitamin E for the average individual."

There is no scientific evidence for this whatever. As a matter of fact every worker who has investigated this particular point has come up with a conclusion which is widely different. Vitamin E, of course, is medical slang and refers to a complex of seven tocopherols, the significant one being *alpha*. It has definitely been established by every worker in the field that the average requirement of alpha tocopherol is 30 international units per day. All sorts of studies made on Dutch and American diets indicate that the average of these diets provides no more than 12 i.u. a day and perhaps much closer to 6 i.u. I don't know how this can be represented as "adequate." In fact, every scientist in the field would say that the average American exists in a chronic state of alpha tocopherol starvation.

The latest of these workers is Horwitt, and it is his work which has recently forced the FDA to revise the statement it has long forced pharmaceutical houses to include in the label of every bottle of Vitamin E [that Vitamin E has not been shown to be necessary in human nutrition]. He showed that since the requirement of alpha tocopherol was 30 i.u. a day, anything less than this tended to haemolyse [destroy] the red blood cells in the human circulation. In other words, intakes averaging less than this jeopardized the red blood cells and human health. This ejected the FDA from the stand they had taken for so many years, but which it should never have taken since Engel and Harris and Quaife had shown at least ten years ago that 30 i.u. was the actual requirement of the human, and had also shown that the average American diet did not have this content. The FDA has been making a serious mistake for the last ten years. It is not its only mistake, and no doubt not its last mistake, but at least a mistake of such dimensions should give you pause before you issue such silly pronouncements as this Service Bulletin contains.

I presume the FDA derives much of its information upon the uselessness of Vitamin E for such diseases as sterility, and so on, heart disease and muscular dystrophy from the American Medical Association. And the American Medical Association has had its problem in this field too. It began by pointing out that about ten years ago there was no evidence that Vitamin E was of value in cardiovascular disease. This was a tremendous mistake, of course. Everyone [except in the United States] now knows that it is very valuable for vascular conditions. Indeed, at the Venice Conference of Vitamin E in 1955 Professor Comel of Italy suggested that the vitamin should henceforth be called the *angiophilic* vitamin because the most outstanding thing about this vitamin was not that it was useful for sterility, but it was useful for vascular conditions of all kinds. There was much evidence for this, of course, when the American Medical Association first began making its derogatory remarks. It is only lately that it has pulled in its horns on vascular disease. Curiously enough, the world medical literature contains some hundreds of useful articles supporting our "wild claims" of 1946 that Vitamin E was useful for heart disease. We continue to wonder how this medical chorus can be overlooked. Surely all of us cannot be wrong. But the American Medical Association can, and it no longer speaks in a derogatory way of the use of vitamin E in vascular disease. I suppose it scarcely could continue to do so ever since recent articles in American medical journals, such as Kawahara (*Surgery* 46:768, 1959).

I intend to go to Washington on January 20th to show how false is the last paragraph in your letter. It shouldn't be hard to do.

I hope that you will have a better understanding of the Vitamin E problem in therapeutics after this note, and I hope that you will be a little slower after this to issue Service Bulletins with factual bases so imperfect.

Sincerely yours,
EVAN V. SHUTE, F.R.C.S.(C)

There is no better illustration of the technique of the Big Lie in orthodox medicine than the foregoing episode. The Better Business Bureau, on medical questions, always assumes the orthodox side, as does Consumers Union. These organizations, in an attempt to "protect" their customers, do not realize that their maintenance of the status quo viewpoint has little validity in many cases. These organizations, should they have existed in Pasteur's time, for instance, would have parroted official medicine's condemnation of Pasteur since he certainly was "outside" orthodox thinking.

The Better Business Bureau, from all my available reports, does an excellent job in its attempt to keep the people informed on shady or outright crooked attempts to fleece the public in matters of confidential schemes or "business" enterprises. In a somewhat comparable field, yet with more technical "testing" of the products, so does Consumers Union. Both these organizations undoubtedly perform a most worthwhile public service. They are both dependent upon member subscriptions for their support and, therefore, are not "official" public agencies. (Neither are the American Medical Association nor the American Cancer Society, though both organizations have achieved that status in the eyes of the American public.)

Yet the Better Business Bureau and Consumers Union have penetrated the fields of science and medicine. Unfortunately, both these organizations have apparently employed medical consultants who are only too happy to rewrite the press releases emanating from Orthodox Headquarters. I receive the same releases and medical news on which the articles are based, and it is exasperating to see two good basic forces in the field of medicine lost to the public because of the seeming inability of the top management to distinguish between clever rewriting of the orthodox handouts and true scientific reporting. Dr. Shute's letter shows us that the fight for science and humanity is still being bitterly resisted by the very "authorities" of the government who should be in the forefront of the battle to protect the people.

No one cognizant of medical history has any illusions about original discoveries throughout the centuries; most were contested unfairly in one way or another. But never before in the relatively short history of civilized man have so many controlling factors been marshaled on the side of the status quo and so few on the side of new discoveries. In almost every field of medical endeavor, orthodox spokesmen, supported or allied with powerful vested interests, have seized such complete control of communications that all attempts by the unorthodox to propose counter and/or advance original theories are ignored or ridiculed; if a controversy reaches the state where it can no longer be ignored or ridiculed, the Big Lie is called into action. The Big Lie when voiced by the proper authorities has seldom failed to achieve its purpose. Book publishing is the last bastion of freedom which we have left. Let us hope we can regain more truth in other areas.

On this rather sombre note we can end our "history" chapter and proceed to other proofs of Vitamin E's efficacy. Let us explore the vitamin's effect on animals.

4

The Animal Evidence

There is so much evidence on various species of animals proving the absolute need of Vitamin E supplementation[16] that one is hardpressed to select and condense it for readers of this book. There are literally thousands of scientific studies, some proving that Vitamin E deficiency will cause heart failure, muscular dystrophy, brain and neurological disorders, reproductive failures, and several other grave ailments which usually prove fatal.

Other studies demonstrate the value of adding Vitamin E to the diet of "normal" animals fed a "normal" diet. Still other experiments prove that Vitamin E will "regenerate" old and aging animals to the point where they are "youthful" again. Indeed, notably in domesticated animals such as dogs, cats, and horses (among others), Vitamin E therapy will "reverse" the aging process for a time. And still other experiments on racing greyhounds and racing horses demonstrate beyond any scientific doubt that the vitamin, when given in adequate dosage, will definitely aid an animal which was already considered to be in superb health or "top form." Human studies bear out the results achieved on animals, as we shall see later.

An important point to remember about animal experimentation is that most of the experiments were "controlled": one group was fed a "normal" diet; another group deprived of Vitamin E; still another received extra supplements of the vitamin. And a most important factor: the animals, of course, did not know they were the subjects of experimentation; they merely

[16] Culik, *et al.;* Curto; Clement; Tolckmitt; Bonadonno and Kaan; Suardi; Gershoff and Norkin; Taylor; Finlaipon and Symons.

ate what was offered them. No doctor put on his best bedside manner and said to the animals: "Now what I'm giving you may help you—it's a new type of therapy." Neither did he look his animal "patients" in the eye and intone hypnotically, "I'm sure you are going to get well. This remedy will work wonders for you."

Anyone who is familiar with medicine knows the "placebo" effect: patients are given harmless, though inactive, pills and, in a controlled study, are compared with patients who are given what purports to be an active remedy. Such is the power of the human mind that the mere thought of receiving benefit enables many of those receiving placebos to get better. Thus, placebos are able to accomplish up to 40 per cent improvement in many illnesses. This strikingly high percentage often approximates the record for the proposed remedy. Sometimes it even surpasses it, if the remedy is toxic and produces harmful side effects. You can see why any medical researcher should be extremely careful in evaluating any new agent on human beings.

However, the placebo effect usually lasts for only a few days, weeks, or possibly months, depending upon the conditions under which the experiment is being conducted. For instance, the placebo improvement almost never continues more than a few days or weeks in the serious illnesses of man such as cancer, heart disease, diabetes, or muscular dystrophy, to mention a few. Yet there is no question that pain—even severe pain such as that experienced in the last stages of some cancers, in tooth extraction, in childbirth, even in major operations—can frequently be eliminated by an expert in hypnosis. In some respects, the process governing the placebo effect is similar to that of hypnosis. In both cases it is the mind of the patient which accomplishes the often astounding results.

With animals, the placebo effect is non-existent, of course. Man has never been able to communicate sufficiently well with the lower species so as to induce the placebo effect as he can in his own more creative and, therefore, imaginative genre. In other words, doctors cannot induce rats, monkeys, dogs, cats, guinea pigs, minks, foxes, cattle, horses, sheep, chickens, and turkeys into thinking they are being helped by supplements of Vitamin E. The objective results are the only elements to reckon with in animal treatments. Some doctors have advanced the hypothesis that Vitamin E produces only a placebo effect in the treatment of human heart disease. (They do not explain the animal results.) Yet there are scores of controlled studies in man, too, which adequately demonstrate that Vitamin E *physiologically,* not psychologically, performs all the essential functions we have reported thus far. But that is for another chapter. For the moment we are concerned with the evidence from our animal friends, which no amount of glib or tortuous reasoning can refute.

We will not go into detail here,[17] but it has been found that healthy rats supplemented with Vitamin E, when compared with healthy rats that were not supplemented, as well as those made deficient in Vitamin E, could swim much longer, could withstand high altitudes 100 per cent better (this experiment was done in a "decompression chamber" such as our astronauts use in training), and could run the "treadmill" longer (a wheel-like device which goes around endlessly as long as the animal or human is able to run).

Further, as even more objective proof, when autopsied after being sacrificed, the Vitamin-E-supplemented rats did not show the same damaging effects on their lungs, kidneys, livers, and other vital organs as did their litter mates who received the same grueling, stressful experiences without Vitamin E supplementation.

Dr. F. Vaccari of Italy has demonstrated that the heart of a frog, when excised from its body and bathed in a solution containing Vitamin E, will beat nearly half again as long as the heart of a frog bathed in normal saline or other nutrient solu-

---

[17] Some of these experiments were conducted by I. R. Telford, *et al.,* at the University School of Aviation Medicine, Randolph Field, Texas. J. Frey and H. Saha are others who found that Vitamin E exerted a most beneficent effect on the hearts and circulatory systems of animals.

tions. The foregoing and other studies show objectively, both in the laboratory and outside it, by testing of performance, that Vitamin E can and does enhance the function of the heart and circulatory system.

We have mentioned Vitamin E deficiencies produced in animals and how they invariably lead to death, preceded, of course, by symptoms which are characteristic of the particular species. The mink, for instance, when fed a diet deficient in Vitamin E, develops what is known as "yellow fat" disease. Before it was discovered that a shortage of Vitamin E was the cause of yellow fat disease, the mortality among mink was enormous. Now, of course, no mink farmer dares *not* to feed his mink extra Vitamin E supplements. (See Benson; and also Van Vliet.) Approximately the same rules of Vitamin E supplementation apply to fox farmers as well.

Raising these animals means quite a bit of money in initial costs and upkeep. And, let us not forget another necessary factor, profit. These animals must have the best in nutrition, and now, thanks to Vitamin E researchers, they get it. Ironically, the farmer himself probably doesn't take the Vitamin E supplement upon which he knows his animals depend for their well being and, in fact, must have in order to produce healthy offspring and to become "marketable" themselves. But the human being is rather slow to learn, particularly if he has been told by an authority that Vitamin E supplements for *him* are absolutely unnecessary. So he dies of a heart attack while feeding his animals the very substance which would have saved his own life!

But minks and foxes are not the only commerically raised animals which need Vitamin E supplementation. You now find the E supplements in chicken and turkey feed. When not fed enough Vitamin E, both these fowls develop peculiarities which lead to their early demise. However, supplements of Vitamin E in their food prevent these diseases, and they are able to bear healthy offspring, which, if Vitamin E-supplemented, will grace your table.

As previously noted, deprivation of E in sheep causes the "stiff-lamb" disease, which means that the lamb dies shortly after birth unless it receives E supplements immediately. Some of the pioneer work on Vitamin-E-deficient lambs and sheep was conducted by F. A. Bacigalupo, R. Culik, *et al.,* and reported in the *Journal of Animal Science* in 1952. (See Bibliography.) Thus, there will be no new generation. Calves born from cows deprived of Vitamin E manifest somewhat the same symptoms. In cattle, the symptoms resemble muscular dystrophy. However, there is little danger now of animals being deprived of an adequate supply of Vitamin E because farmers and the pharmaceutical houses have been alerted to the danger.

Now, let us consider old dogs and cats. For our evidence here, among others, we have N. H. Lambert, a famous veterinarian of Dublin, who is a Fellow of the Royal College of Veterinary Surgeons, a title not perfunctorily granted. Dr. Lambert's other credits are many and varied, for his special talent seems to be the capacity for original thinking and the willingness to experiment no matter what the opposition.

He had read of Dr. Shute's work in Canada on humans; forthwith, he resolved to test Vitamin E on some of his old dog "heart patients." His very first case treated with Vitamin E astounded both Dr. Lambert (who was prepared for a favorable effect) and the owner of the dog. Shortened, Dr. Lambert's report reads: "An eleven-year-old Griffon bitch in very poor physical condition [after the usual conventional treatments] . . . the heart was rapidly deteriorating. The owner implored me to do anything to save the bitch's life. At this stage she was having frequent heart attacks, was very wasted, was almost too weak to stand, and had to be hand-fed with liquids." Vitamin E was administered, 3 I.U. three times a day. "After the first day, a slight improvement was noticed; this improvement was maintained and in fourteen days the dog was moving around, barking, and actually looking for food. The result was spectacular, and her owner stated two months later that she was younger in her ways than [she had been] for the past three years. Nearly twelve months after treatment started, she played like a pup, had a fine glossy coat, and had her first normal heat in four years, followed by a phantom pregnancy!" Phantom pregnancy approximates a "false" or pseudo-pregnancy in the human; that is, some of the signs and symptoms of pregnancy are present, except for the actual existence of the foetus in the womb. This dog enjoyed "excellent health" for several more years, until finally old age overtook her as it customarily does with every living creature. Her owner then reluctantly requested euthanasia.

Dr. Lambert's second case was a twelve-year-old fox terrier. The symptoms were coughing and a disinclination to go for walks. The terrier was very weak and refused all food. Dr. Lambert's examination revealed endocarditis (inflammation of the lining membrane of the heart) and heart dilation. The dog was given 3 I.U. of Vitamin E three times a day to start. It improved slowly, according to Dr. Lambert's reports; the owner later noted it was "rejuvenated and played again like a pup."

The third case offered here—an eight-year-old Red Setter—is a fitting tribute to most men's ignorance of how a natural remedy should and ought to function, an ignorance fostered by the orthodox who think that if a remedy works, it should be stopped when the patient gets better.

This dog had a large *adenoma* (tumor) of the anus which was being partially regressed by administration of a synthetic female hormone. (Often in the human, treatments with hormones of the opposite sex will temporarily regress a cancer in the sexual regions. For instance, males with cancer of the prostrate gland will frequently obtain relief through administration of the female hormone, estrogen.)

But the owner of this dog was taking him out regularly for hunting, which some animal lovers may consider reprehensible, since the owner was aware of the dog's serious condition. However, six weeks later, the dog was brought in again. He had collapsed several times while hunting, and when seen the second time by Dr. Lambert, he was "very wasted, with laboured breathing, and coughing a great deal." Dr. Lambert's examination demonstrated "advanced endocarditis and cardiac dilation," which proves what a dog will do for his master.

He was treated with Vitamin E. "An immediate improvement was noticed by the owner, and as little as a week later, the dog . . . was in good form and breathing normally." Dr. Lambert advised gradual increase of diet and exercise. Hunting, naturally, was forbidden. However, three weeks later, when the irrepressible hunter returned with his dog, he related he had just returned from giving the dog "a three-days shooting" and that he was "nearly as good as ever."

As Dr. Lambert states rather scientifically, although we can note his disapproval between the lines, "the owner put the dog through a regular hunting season, giving him Vitamin E, when he appeared tired." The next season, the hunter did not give the dog any Vitamin E. It is not surprising that halfway through the hunting season, the old, faithful dog dropped dead in "the middle of the second day's shoot."

Although Dr. Lambert has scores of cases similar to the aforementioned, we must content ourselves with two more examples.

A sixteen-year-old neutered cat had collapsed with a heart attack and, when seen by Dr. Lambert, had a very rapid and weak pulse. It could not walk straight. After Vitamin E therapy, however, this old cat made what most would call a "miraculous" recovery. It developed "kittenish" habits and looked younger than it had five years before.

The following case is also most significant, especially if one is interested in racing. The owner of a twenty-months-old racing greyhound came to Dr. Lambert. The dog had won its first 525-yard race in 30.9 seconds. However, following this race it dwindled away, condition and energy gone. It was rested for a month, but this usual procedure had little beneficent effect. It just stopped before the finish line in its next race. It was then rested for two months. In another race in which it was finally tried, it stopped at 300 yards and pitifully *crawled* to the finish tape. This act of courage revealed its fighting spirit, as well as its ill health.

When it was brought to Dr. Lambert's clinic, the greyhound was immediately diagnosed as a heart disease case and put on Vitamin E therapy. To quote the exact words of Dr. Lambert: "He improved beyond belief and has since won seven races, is very fit and the heart appears normal."

And have you read about the "brave bulls" which are supposed to charge the men opposing them until they are dispatched in the so-called, much-publicized "moment of truth"? There are, of course, many bulls that are sacrificed in this fashion in the Spanish bull rings every year. Yet who is aware that many bulls, in spite of their deliberately inbred and carefully fostered hatred of man, really cannot perform properly in the arena due to a lack of Vitamin E?

Many bulls who apparently would like to gore their tormentors cannot do so because they fall down in the fight before being killed by the gracefully performing matador or his cohorts. They are victims of what we call either "strokes" or "heart failures" in humans. Yet even after their seizures, some try nobly to perform their set roles in the drama of the bullfight, but usually they are unable to carry on; in the end, all are knifed and wheeled away, classified as cowards by the watching humans, who would think themselves extraordinarily courageous if *they* could, after suffering a heart attack, stagger to the nearest telephone or doctor's office. Now, however, we have the benefit of some Spanish investigators who have determined the cause for the failure of some bulls to continue performing in the ring. Dr. D. Jordano and Dr. C. Gaspar Gomez studied 513 bulls who fell in the ring before they could be killed. They concluded that the circulatory and central nervous systems were drastically affected and that there was a "direct relationship between this condition and Vitamin-E deficiency." (See also Bonadonna and Kaan.)

Let us now examine horse racing. When we say horse racing,

we also include horse breeding. These are the two factors with which we are concerned. The original experiments with Vitamin E in horse racing and horse breeding were undertaken at the Windfields Farm, Toronto, Canada, and the National Stud Farm in Oshawa, Canada. The owner of both farms, E. P. Taylor, offered his entire stock of thoroughbred racers for the experiment with Vitamin E. The plan for the experiment was devised by Dr. Evan Shute and William Jay Gutterson, President of Webber Pharmaceuticals, Limited, Toronto, Canada, which organization supplied the Vitamin E. The report on the results of a two-year-study was issued by F. G. Darlington, manager of the farms and the experiment, and J. B. Chassels, a Doctor of Veterinary Medicine, both of whom supervised the experiments.

The farm began its study of Vitamin E supplementation midway in the racing season of 1955. All concerned were so impressed with the results that the study was continued into the following year (and, of course, continues to the present day, but we are now dealing with the original experiments). The authors of the study put the problem very practically. In fact the subtitle of one of their papers is termed quite appropriately: "Practical Aspects of a Racing Study." The authors state:

The successful operation of a racing stable depends on consistency of performance. An owner is vitally interested in the number of races per start that is won. If horses are not winning, it is of paramount importance that they be in the money a good percentage of the time, since second and third monies sometimes contribute 50 per cent of a stable's earnings. In Canada, a racing stable must win an average of two and a half races per horse per year in order to break even, and its horses should be in the money at least one-third of the times they run.

As you know, horse racing is a business as well as a sport. This means no nonsense or crackpot schemes are tolerated. Nothing matters which does not ring the cash register enough to warrant a continuance of the methods employed in the business-sport.

I quote from the summary of the Darlington-Chassels Report: "The percentage of wins per horse was 2.7 (cf. 2.3 last year [when the Vitamin E experiment began] and 1.8 in 1954, the year before the tocopherol experiment began)." Thus we see that the percentage of wins increased approximately two-thirds under Vitamin E supplementation.

Further, the farm found that, although the percentage of wins per horse jumped from 1.8 to 2.3 in the first year of Vitamin E supplementation, the horses hit their peak of efficiency the following year when their dosages were doubled or tripled. The horses' earnings, where the same horses were compared in the two years, also increased approximately two-thirds on the larger dose—$46,405 vs. $76,410, to be exact. Remember this is a comparison between *small* and *large* doses of Vitamin E, *not* among animals not receiving it at all.

In 1956, having increased the number of animals taking Vitamin E, the farm's actual take was $196,685 vs. $88,260 the previous year. The number of winners was 95 compared with 80. The number of seconds ("place") increased from 25 to 40, and the number of third running horses ("show") increased from 17 to 30.

These are the cold, hard, cash facts. Not only did the farm ascertain that Vitamin E improved its earnings very considerably, but there were many other favorable aspects. Race horses are notoriously "high-strung"; and some refuse to eat properly. The trainers found that under Vitamin E therapy almost all of these "too-nervous" horses were gradually quieted and began normal feeding, concomitant with their greatly improved performances on the track. (This calming effect was first discovered on human beings by German researchers, who called Vitamin E, "nature's own tranquilizer.")

Let us now take a couple of typical examples of how Vitamin E worked in the equine racing experiment. Listed in the report is horse #12, a stallion six years old. As the report points out, most race horses have passed their peak at that age. Two years previously, as a four-year-old and before receiving Vitamin E, #12 made twelve starts, winning one race, coming in second in another, and third in still another. His earnings that year were $2,595, his average per race being $216. On April 10, 1955, #12 began receiving 800 units of Vitamin E daily. On August 15, this dose was increased to 2,000 units. That season, the horse made fourteen starts, winning five times, "placing" three times, and "showing" once. His earnings jumped to $10,090, his average per race being $721.

By that time the experimenters had decided that Vitamin E should be maintained all during the year, not just during the racing season: accordingly #12 was placed on a 1,000 unit dosage daily during the winter. At the start of the racing season of 1956, this dosage was increased to 2,000 units daily. In that year, when the horse should have been giving signs of "slipping" and his owners should have been thinking about putting him out to stud, he *made his best record*. In thirteen starts, he won five, "placed" in three, and "showed" once. His earnings were $13,355, and his average per race was $1,027. On the record, this appears approximately similar to the preceding year. But #12 showed more stamina and ran better and faster than the preceding year. According to the report, on one occasion he established a new track record! Most significantly, in five of six races *throughout the year* there was not three fifths of a second's difference in his time. The "old hoss" showed what he was made of and what could be done, abetted of course with Vitamin E. He, like every horse in the stable, was given a double dose of Vitamin E prior to each race. And often, on the morning of the race, the racers were again given a double dose to increase muscular stamina and utilization of oxygen.

As for the "nervous" and "poor feeding" horses, the Darlington-Chassels Report states: ". . . the first week we gave 5,000 units daily, the second week 3,000 units, afterward 2,000. We had three horses where this regime was not entirely successful; in each of these cases we went back to the higher dosage and started over again. *We did not have a failure finally.*" (Emphasis mine.)

There are many such examples of a Vitamin E-supplemented horse "coming back" or exceeding what he or she ever did. In fact, as if we needed more proof, during the racing season, Vitamin E was cut down or out and then reinstituted. *The performance of the horse directly followed the pattern of the Vitamin E intake.* For scientists and anyone else, I recommend a complete perusal of the Darlington-Chassels Report which is available in the December, 1956, *Summary.*

A word of caution, however. Vitamin E will never make a winner out of a "plug." It can never take the place of heredity, a good diet, and excellent training. When an athlete competes (and the horse is certainly an athlete), he must be at the top of his form. Vitamin E increases his capacity even when he is considered in "top form." (This, of course, does not mean that Vitamin E will not benefit those organisms—human or horses—which are not in top shape. It means merely that in any competitive endeavor, athletes must be at their best. Vitamin E makes them "better than best.")

Of course, there are many questions which were asked about Vitamin E's effectiveness in horse racing. Most, as may be expected, came from owners and trainers of racehorses. Chief among these questions: What is the exact way in which alpha tocopherol (Vitamin E) brings about these helpful changes in the body of a racehorse? Answer, Darlington-Chassels Report:

It enables the tissues of the body to do the same job on less oxygen; it is as if one strapped an aqua-lung [with oxygen] on the horse's back. It opens up huge reserves of capillary circulation, sets of vessels not ordinarily used but waiting there for emergency demands. It helps to control the passage of fluids through the walls of blood vessels. It may even be a direct stimulant of muscle power. It improves the metabolism of carbohydrates, fats, and proteins. These are just a few of its unique and helpful properties.

Q. How much do horses improve? [With Vitamin E therapy]

A. The degree of improvement that does take place depends entirely upon the class of animal being worked with. In a general way, it will bring horses close to their best effort, provided their physical condition and soundness are in good order.

Q. Have you had corroborative reports from other owners and trainers?

A. Yes, we have had many but not as many and of the type we would like to have. [Here are scientists speaking who want experiments performed in the completely objective, scientific manner in which the Darlington-Chassels study was done.] The reason for this seems to be that if an alpha-tocopherol-treated horse does improve, its owner or trainer wants to take the credit.

Q. Are you continuing the experiments?

A. Of course . . . some very interesting avenues have been opened up through some of our inquiries and a great deal of work is now under way in some of the leading universities in America. . . .

Unfortunately, the time lag between medical findings and their reaching the general public is so long that it may be quite some time before these results are made available. Vitamin E, of course, is not classified by any government as a drug or narcotic. But it also is not recognized by official medical agencies that the vitamin will produce any extra benefits on either animals or men, even if they take more than the minimum daily requirement as suggested by the National Research Council. As we have mentioned, it is the pharmacological effect of massive dosages which produces the beneficial results noted here; its action is then as a drug or a medicine, not a vitamin *per se*. In the human, in the U.S., the minimum daily requirement happens to be set at six units a day, a ridiculously low figure, as we have seen in Dr. Shute's letter in Chapter 3.

Another report, issued by Darlington-Chassels covering five years instead of two, appears in *The Summary,* Dec., 1960. The report confirms the original findings, but most of this later study was devoted to the breeding of thoroughbreds rather than to racing. We shall examine this report shortly. However, in a summary of their findings, Darlington-Chassels state rather tersely: "The performance of the racehorses of this stable reached a new high in Canada during the progress of this study."

Indeed, they did. For instance, according to the Report, the "best horse ever sired in Canada, Victoria Park, was by

Chop Chop, the oldest stud, when he was 16." Chop Chop as well as Victoria Park's mother, received ample supplies of Vitamin E before he [Victoria Park] was conceived, and he was trained and raced under Vitamin E therapy. He was declared "Horse of the Year" in Canada in 1960 after winning $250,076. He had placed third in the Kentucky Derby. However, an accident prevented his continuing his most promising racing career and he was retired to stud at the age of three, just when most colts are beginning their careers.

Probably the most dramatic Vitamin E-bred and trained horse is Northern Dancer, the little three-year-old colt who was offered for sale two years ago for $25,000 with no takers. To date, Northern Dancer has earned close to $2,000,000, winning the Kentucky Derby and the Preakness and placing third in the Belmont. The little Vitamin E-sired and trained horse has won 14 out of 17 starts and has never finished out of the money.

In the past five years, tocopherol-bred horses have won the "Queen's Plate," a racing event in Canada comparable to the Kentucky Derby in the U.S. The proud owner, E. P. Taylor, was recently quoted in *Fortune* magazine as saying "I only like winners." Mr. Taylor is probably one of the wealthiest men in the world, and this fortune was largely accumulated through his own ingenuity and skill; competition being what it is, can one blame Mr. Taylor for not announcing at the Kentucky Derby and the Preakness that his horses had increased their winnings by two-thirds just by the ingestion of Vitamin E?

However, there is more information available about the vitamin's uses other than improving the performances of race horses, their eating habits, and their generally nervous dispositions. The National Stud Farm also provides us with thorough documentation concerning the effects of the vitamin in breeding mares, stallions, and even geldings, which are not supposed to have an interest in females, having been relieved of the organs necessary for sexual activity and procreation.

There have been hundreds of studies done on other animals in various laboratories throughout the world, all of which have proven that Vitamin E is indeed a "rejuvenator" in the sexual aspect. However, many researchers think its role in the sexual realm is purely the result of having built up the body to such a state of health that it is naturally reflected in sexual activity. Be that as it may, the fact is Vitamin E works, not only on horses but other animals as well. (We shall examine the role of Vitamin E's efficiency on man's fertility later.) To mention a few who have been responsible for the fertility findings in animals: Dr. A. Bonfert and Dr. J. Arp (Germany); Dr. A. M. Brown, Dr. M. J. Cook, Dr. W. Lane-Petter, Dr. G. Porter, and Dr. A. A. Tuffery (England); Dr. Barbaro D'Agostino (Milan, Italy); as well as hundreds of others listed in the *Annotated Bibliography of Vitamin E, 1958–1960.*

Since our primary interest in this chapter is animal evidence, we shall return to the horse experiment. (Because of lack of space, we cannot cite all the animal references, but we refer the interested reader to the Bibliography.) The Darlington-Chassels Report was motivated not only by the scientific desire for learning but also by financial considerations; it was concerned with how much gain there was in Vitamin E for the National Stud Farm. We are sure that every word of the report is true not only in the scientific sense, but also in the economic sphere. The report was entitled *Breeding Experiments in 1956.* The subtitle, as we might suppose, is termed *General Economic Considerations.*

In a preliminary statement, which takes us to the crux of the problem, the report states:

The owners of thoroughbred brood mares and stallions are vitally interested in the number of registered foals that can be produced. For the market breeder this can mean the difference between his farm's profit and loss. . . . Obviously both time and money can be saved if the fertility of his animals is increased.

It would be impossible to estimate accurately in dollars what could be saved if only a 5 per cent increase in fertility was achieved. There are literally millions of dollars involved. Neither would it be possible to estimate what it could mean in perpetuating some great line or in the production of the occasional great horse, which otherwise might never be born.

Veterinarians and farm managers focus their primary interest on conception. If the percentage of pregnancies can be raised, it will automatically mean a higher number of living and registered foals. . . . Tables giving data from conception to foaling to registration have been worked out, and [from them we see] that there is nearly a fixed percentage of loss to be expected during pregnancy and at delivery. The prime key to success, therefore, is attention paid to sire and mare before and at breeding time. At the National Stud Farm all our research is directed at that source of success, which is conception. . . . In our initial Report, we were able to report only definite pregnancies and anticipated foals, but now, *after* two breeding seasons, we are able to demonstrate the result of our studies in actual foal registration. . . .

We cannot present the whole report here. But we can, at least, reprint the Introduction which we might consider a classic in practicality.

In the operation of a breeding farm it is a well known fact that there is very little if any profit from boarding revenue. It depends upon stud fees to make a showing on the right side of the ledger. While a 5 per cent increase in conceptions may seem insignificant to uninformed persons, it must be remembered that valuable stallions demand stud fees up to $10,000 and their progeny as yearlings will bring up to $50,000. Thus, a 5 per cent improved fertility in a stud standing for $4,000 and bred to one hundred mares over a three-year period would mean another $25,000 to the owner.

To accomplish even slight increases in impregnation, a stallion must be working at optimum. His success or failure as a sire depends upon the number of progeny he gets to the races. His value in dollars and cents to his owner is dependent upon the number of mares he is capable of handling in a season, how great a percentage of these he is able to get in foal, and how readily conception occurs.

It has been the practice on large breeding farms owning valuable sires strictly to limit the number of covers a stallion makes per season in order to preserve his usefulness. Many times a valuable stud fee and one year of a mare's fertile life are wasted through this procedure. Our experience with stallions given Vitamin E has been that now we can get those essential extra covers. In the past we had tried to keep down to an average of two services per mare. In the 1956 season we had an average of slightly more than three —yet our stallions came through the season in fine condition.

The summary of the experiment, very much oversimplified, is somewhat the following: the experimenters used every type of mare from the old barren ones to the two-year-old fillies. They also utilized old stallions long past their day as "controls"; they used medium-aged stallions as well as young ones filled with what we may term intensely driving sexual impulses. And as the experimenters state: exactly the same methods of breeding were maintained with Vitamin E as before, the same amount of what is called "teasing" and being placed in close proximity.

Now, the Jockey Club, the apparent authority in the racing field, says that pregnant mares can be expected to produce registered foals 52 per cent of the time. Yet under Vitamin E therapy for both stallions and mares, the National Stud Farm was able to achieve 71 per cent registered foals, truly a significant increase when all of the old mares, the erstwhile barren mares, and the old stallions are taken into consideration. The percentage would have been undoubtedly higher had only the younger horses been included in the experiment. But as it is, I think any dispassionate scientist would agree the old horses did very well indeed.

As stated in the Darlington-Chassels Report:

Alpha tocopherol . . . illustrates clearly that this agent improves the fertility of both mares and stallions. . . . In this year's experiment 88 per cent of 18 barren mares, 100 per cent of 6 maiden mares, and 84 per cent of 31 foaling mares conceived. . . . Stallions taking alpha tocopherol continued to behave and perform better in general. . . . From five stallions on Vitamin E, at least 71 per cent of registered foals are anticipated this year— 8 per cent above *their* [own] average for the preceding five years.

In the five-year report, we will only quote the summary concerning fertility since it merely corroborates the earlier findings: "Alpha tocopherol (Vitamin E) in proper dosage improved the fertility of mares and stallions, this being most evident in the older animals."

Need we say any more about animals and their benefit from Vitamin E? There is much more material available on animals besides the evidence presented here. I have tried to list some of the most significant references in the Bibliography. One cannot ignore the overwhelming evidence on animals, especially when it is correlated with all the evidence we know about humans.

When I was still in the sceptical stage about the value of Vitamin E, I made a personal determination for myself. A fourteen-year-old cat, named Old Tom, which lived next door to me, used to be the terror of the neighborhood. Wherever he went, the other cats moved aside. Females that were in heat, of course, were excepted. In fact, Tom forced many a powerful male cat to move from the neighborhood because he established precedence over the females (and males) and would not tolerate any other males which might seek to share *affaires d'amour* with his many lady loves.

In battle with other males, Tom had no match. In fact, even dogs were afraid of him. Some did test his fighting prowess at first, but as he was not only powerful but ingenious, he gained a most respectable reputation, even among dogs. Thus, he ruled the neighborhood for twelve years, which brings us to the point of this passage. Old Tom suddenly began to fail. It was almost unbelievable at the beginning. First, the sexual impulses diminished to the point where he could look at a female cat in heat without displaying the slightest reaction. Then all the male cats in the neighborhood which he had intimidated and/or beaten (including two of ours) began to take certain liberties. They would jump in his yard and some would even steal his food, to which atrocious actions he offered not the slightest objection. He would just sit in the sun and ignore everything.

However, since his owner had to be away from home frequently, Old Tom did not receive his food as regularly as he would have wished. He began frequenting our house, and my wife could not resist feeding him. But she found that his whole attitude had changed. Before, he had been a bristling, belligerent animal, hostile to almost anyone and everything. Now he was a whining, crawling beggar. He did not show any hostility when our cats would hiss and growl at him. He was completely subdued by life, or if we wish to put it bluntly, he was subdued and cowed by old age. There was nothing left for him to do but die or beg.

To put Vitamin E to another test, I added 50 I.U. daily to Old Tom's diet. The results would amaze someone who knew nothing about Vitamin E's action. Within a week, Old Tom began to take an extremely renewed interest in life. He savagely mauled the various cats who thought he was done for (including one of ours); he pursued the female cats who were in heat (there were several), but most significant of all to me, his pride came back. He stopped begging food from us. Prior to Vitamin E in massive doses, he would look at us and immediately his mouth would fly open in an automatic wail—the cat had no pride. Now, under Vitamin E, his pride had returned. However, since he had mauled one of our cats and was attempting to drive them away as is the custom of the species, we decided not to give Old Tom any more Vitamin E.

The effect, after about two weeks, was almost as miraculous as the previous experiment. Old Tom returned to his old senile patterns and now is on good terms with our cats and all cats, without sex, without any drive except for food and perhaps some petting. But he wails at us day and night, helpless, and without pride, waiting for death without knowing it.

Let us hope we never have to encounter death in that fashion; I do not believe we will if Vitamin E and other nutrients are utilized in the proper fashion. There is no question but that every animal and every man has to die; yet life might be preserved, more abundantly, in full vigor, for much longer had we the wisdom to apply the findings already known about Vitamin E.

5

Heart Disease Evidence

Now that we have introduced the reader to the fundamental information about Vitamin E, its long and documented history, and the evidence from animals which supports its effectiveness, we turn to the crucial material which most directly affects the human being.

Almost everyone who can read or watch television or listen to the radio knows that heart disease, along with associated circulatory disorders, is America's number one killer; that diseases of the cardiovascular system account for more than four times as many victims as the next leading cause of death, cancer; that there are between 11,000,000 and 12,000,000 sufferers from heart ailments; that more than half the men over forty-five die from coronary thrombosis; that more women, especially over forty-five, are succumbing to heart maladies; and that these disorders are reaching deeper into the ranks of younger persons.

An interesting observation about this last fact is that, of those soldiers killed in the Korean War who were autopsied, an astounding 77 per cent showed evidence of blood vessels that were "hardened" or "thickened," clogged up by fatty deposits; these men, undoubtedly, would have been candidates for coronary attacks had they lived. The average age of these soldiers was *only 22!* No one can very well assert that a "soft life" and "lack of exercise" initiated this condition. The soldiers' training was tough and rigorous, and their everyday existence under total war was even tougher. It was so tough in fact that it cost them their lives.

Was it tension, then, that laid down the ominous arteriosclerotic *plaques* on the linings of their blood vessels? As we know, tension and modern living have been blamed for the tremendous increase in heart disease. In World Wars I and II, many thousands of soldiers were autopsied. They were just as subject to tension and worry as those in Korea. Isn't it logical to assume that if medical men had found the same startling evidence of incipient cardiovascular disease, they would have made the fact known? In an Army (or any other) autopsy, everything that is found is reported. That is the purpose of a "general" autopsy. The doctors performing the Korean autopsies were not looking for anything in particular. They just reported what they found, as did the doctors in World Wars I and II. In order not to confuse the reader by presenting seemingly contradictory statements, may I say that I found no evidence explaining why the World Wars I and II soldiers evidently did not have nascent cardiovascular conditions such as the Korean soldiers had. This is a problem which should be investigated by reputable researchers.

Animal fats in the American diet have been blamed as a chief cause of arterial "clogging." Yet, as any GI will tell you, his diet, for the most part, was not abundant in fats. In fact, in most front lines the diet was hardly adequate. Besides, exercise is supposed to counteract some of the evils fats are hypothesized to do within the human body; indeed, exercise *is* helpful in metabolizing fat.

Could the puzzle be related to the diet in a way which almost no one has thought about? Could it be a *deficiency* which is afflicting not only the GI, but a majority of the American people, a growing, creeping type of deficiency which no one ever suspected?

Daily, we are inundated by authoritarian opinions that animal fats in our diet are largely responsible for our consistently rising heart attack toll. Now that other evidence has been brought out, the authoritarian anti-cholesterol, anti-fat crusade has wavered considerably. At the moment, authorities are conceding there is no simple answer to the riddle of heart disease.

We have presented other evidence in support of this fact, but a recent scientific study of the Samburu, a tribe in North Kenya, offers another truly puzzling question. The Samburu keep herds of sheep and goats which they treasure very highly since they live almost entirely on the milk of the animals—no vegetables, fruits, or grains, except for an occasional tuber. They drink the milk of the animals and periodically bleed them and drink the raw blood—something which seems repugnant to our taste. They eat the flesh of their animals, but this is not too often, for instinctively they know well the old adage "Don't kill the goose that laid the golden egg." But, ironically, the seemingly undernourished Samburu get more Vitamin E from their simple diet of milk, meat, and blood than we get from our "affluent" diet.

The scientific team of Dr. Shaper and Dr. Jones, who made the study of the Samburu tribe as reported in *Lancet* (1962), was amazed that while about *60 per cent* of these peoples' total calories are derived from animal fats found in the milk, yet a check of their blood revealed that it was *low in fatty materials*. As if to confute the "high-fat-always-equals-heart-disease" hypothesis further, heart disease and associated concomitants such as high blood pressure were practically unknown among the Samburu.

And they do not, apparently, have a high death rate since there are many old persons in the tribe. The research team ran electrocardiograms on one hundred of these elderly persons. They found only two of them who might possibly have a suggestion of cardiovascular trouble, but even these were not confirmed clinically. In other words, there were no physical complaints.

There may be those who say then that exercise is the key and that that is why the Samburu have no heart disease and *we* have so much. Yet there are many tribes and cultures all over the world which exercise fully as much as the Samburu and some of them have heart disease.

It is a pity that the white man destroyed the original Esquimo culture along with his original diet before a thoroughly scientific study was possible. However, we do know what the Esquimos ate; we also know their way of life as ascertained by several early explorers. Several researchers feel that the Esquimos were comparable with the present-day Samburu, though the Esquimos lived in the frozen Arctic while the Samburu still live in the heart of Africa—totally different environments—yet each existing entirely on animals and animal products. The Esquimos ate the whole animal, fat and blubber included, as well as organs, muscles, connective tissue such as cartilage, and bone marrow, without *any* vegetables, fruits, or grains, until the white man came in with his civilized diet and germs.

The great scholarly Arctic explorer, the late Vilhjalmur Stefansson, author of many reputable books, compiled from existing records a remarkable account of the ancient Esquimos and compared them with "modern" man (*My Life with the Eskimo* and *Cancer: Disease of Civilization?*). His evidence strongly corroborates the validity of the hypothesis that raw animal products (which contain generous amounts of Vitamin E) may be man's natural food, protecting him from the various diseases of so-called civilization. The aboriginal Esquimos were not victims of cancer, heart disease, or tuberculosis, even though many apparently lived to be quite old, according to the early traders.

Stefansson was unable to study the Esquimo in his pristine state because, by the time he arrived on the scene, the white man's diseases had taken such a toll of the Esquimo that it was only the toughest of them who were able to survive at all. Almost all of their progeny had been so over-awed by the white man's technology that they assumed he also knew about nutrition; therefore, white sugar and white flour (with practically all the nutrients, including Vitamin E, processed out) became prize commodities in Esquimo homes as a mark of prestige. Wouldn't any race which could fly through the air, build huge ships that traversed the seas, and shoot a polar bear at a distance of 400 yards—would not this race know best how to eat also? The idea was laughable that a race who could accomplish what the gods had not accomplished before would not know healthy living. So the Esquimos died by the thousands from various germs and those who survived became victims of tooth decay, heart disease, cancer, and the various diseases which afflict the white man.

The same situation prevailed for the American Indian. Of course, no one became really interested in studying him until it was too late to obtain clear-cut, definite results which science would accept. However, the Samburu study is most significant. It may be even more so when they stop drinking milk and blood after accepting our standards for a "well-nourished" diet.

As the reader may know, almost everything—from lack of proteins, to lack of exercise, to too much animal fats, to the pace of modern living—has been blamed for the phenomenal increase in heart disease. We have put on record that none of these is the sole cause of heart disease. The following offers some additional proof that no single factor as previously postulated is responsible.

In World War II, doctors were assigned to study the condition of the prisoners at Dachau,[18] one of the most infamous of the Nazi concentration camps. As pictures from this camp reveal, the pitiful condition of most of the inmates would lead no one to say the prisoners were over-fed. In fact, as captured documents testify, these human beings were being starved to death. Also, in addition to the Jews, there were a number of political prisoners, which makes the following study even more scientific than if it had been based solely upon one particular group.

The doctors autopsied 10,000 inmates of Dachau, who were victims of mass executions or epidemics. They did not have to estimate the number of calories each inmate received since the Nazis were very careful bookkeepers. An amazing concept to our minds, they kept the records until almost the day they were

[18] See Bibliography: *Journal American Geriatric Society.*

overwhelmed by the Allies. Therefore, we know that each inmate of their *conzentrazion-slager* received an average of 1,000 calories per day. (Toward the end of the war this ration was cut to 500 calories.) We also know how those calories were dispersed. The inmates were fed daily a mixture of weak soup and a slice of black bread. There was very little protein or fats, mostly carbohydrates. Of course, we must remember that on a starvation or semi-starvation diet, a person uses his own reserves of fats, proteins, minerals, and vitamins until his body reservoirs are depleted, usually within a month or six weeks. The inmates could not be expected to survive for long on such meager fare, especially since they were forced to perform hard physical labor every day. Yet it is a significant fact that none of the prisoners complained of heart symptoms, and so far as is known, none *died* of cardiovascular disease. But most significant and astounding of all is the fact that every one of the 10,000 autopsied showed evidence of arteriosclerosis! Now this pattern was repeated throughout the world where there were prisoners. Men, even on the horrible fare served to them in prison camps, do not *die* of heart disease. They may starve to death as often happened, but their hearts and cardiovascular systems are apparently intact enough to sustain them for a time and are not the direct cause of death.

Could the black bread the prisoners received have contained enough Vitamin E to prevent the overt *symptoms* of arteriosclerosis in a steadily deteriorating body? Perhaps. Another significant finding was that almost none of the prisoners suffered from high blood pressure—a frequent concomitant of arteriosclerosis. This may be one reason why the prisoners did not suffer from the usual results of arteriosclerosis: "stroke," coronaries, etc. The editors of the *Journal of the American Geriatric Society* have suggested that "mental stress" was a large factor in producing the universal arteriosclerosis at Dachau. This may well be, but we have seen that tension and stress alone cannot account for all arteriosclerosis. And who is to explain the lack of high blood pressure, which is supposed to be a partial result of stress and/or tension? Of course, we must admit that had the prisoners lived long enough, there might have been a high incidence of deaths from cardiovascular disease.

Thus, we see almost every explanation offered as the *cause* of cardiovascular diseases has large loop-holes and contradictory evidence.

Let us examine more of the hypotheses.

Lest anyone think that a vegetarian diet (either self-imposed or occurring naturally) will protect him from cardiovascular troubles, he should heed the several scientific observations on both man and animals which disprove this notion. Scientific advocates of the hypothesis that animal fat is the sole cause of cardiovascular diseases have found ardent champions in the vegetarian groups. Since they have long advocated that *raw* (sometimes cooked) vegetables and grains *alone* will prevent or cure heart diseases, among other ailments, it may be apropos to examine some of the evidence.

Such groups are fond of quoting the fact that vegetarian animals living in the wild, natural state would almost never die if they were not victims of accidents: disasters such as being eaten by a carnivore or shot by man. These groups thus imply that man, being an animal, would be able to achieve near-immortal status physically if he refrained from ingesting other animals.

No doubt there is a good deal to be said in favor of raw, fresh vegetables as an adjunct to man's diet. Man is an omnivore, as indicated by the length of his intestine. The carnivores possess a short intestine while the herbivores, having to break down plants for nutrition, have a very long intestine because the breakdown is more complicated. Man, along with bears and rats, is endowed with a medium-length intestine, capable of digesting both plant and animal food. But man is probably more carnivorous than vegetarian, as he can live healthily on raw animal products while it has never been shown that he can live healthily purely on vegetables and fruits. (Even the most famous vegetarian of them all, George Bernard Shaw, took liver extract.) Eggs, milk, and cheese are, of course, animal products. If man cannot eat the whole animal raw, as the carnivores do (and to some extent the Samburu and the original Esquimos), then he should supplement his diet with fruits and vegetables, preferably in the natural state. (Of course carnivores and the groups of men we have mentioned grow old and die, but probably not specifically of heart diseases.)

The studies that have been made on wild vegetarian animals have necessarily been limited, but they are extremely meaningful. They confirm that these animals do suffer and undoubtedly do die from cardiovascular disorders remarkably similar to those of "civilized" man. The latest of these studies was reported by Dr. B. McKinney in 1962, in *Lancet,* a leading medical journal in Britain. His work was done in Uganda on the buffalo, the hippopotamus, and the wild cow. Now, these animals would starve to death rather than eat a piece of meat. Even if meat were rammed down their throats, they would not be able to digest it as their digestive organs are geared only for vegetable consumption.

Yet Dr. McKinney found "fatty streaks" in their aortas "similar to those in man." Under the microscope, these arteriosclerotic plaques in the heart vessels "closely" resembled those in humans in that there was thickening of the arterial walls, fibrosis, and fatty material in the lining of the walls. It was obvious that the fatty materials in the arterial walls were formed from the carbohydrate material which the animals ate exclusively.

As if we needed more proof that the causal relationship of heart disease and related symptoms is not due to a low animal fat diet, "tension," or other such factors, it is afforded to us in abundance by Drs. McCullagh, Perry, and Lewis writing in the *New England Journal of Medicine* in 1960 (see Bibliography).

The doctors studied Trappist monks, who are noted for their placid life (free of everyday tension) and their abstinence from all animal foods except milk and a small amount of cheese. Their diet was extremely low in animal fats, containing only about 36 grams of butterfats per day; yet the monks ate a moderate amount of the "unsaturated fatty acids." And their average serum cholesterol *was* a bit lower than a group of Cleveland businessmen of the same age. (This finding is important when we realize that a low-animal fat diet is believed by some researchers not only to bring the blood cholesterol down, but in turn to prevent arteriosclerosis and, therefore, heart attacks, strokes, and associated cardiovascular disorders.)

Yet on examination of forty-four monks over the age of forty, the researchers found that some "retinal vascular disease" was evident in 59 per cent, and "some degree of hypertension" (high blood pressure) was present in 48 per cent of these monks. The authors noted that high blood pressure "is more frequent [in the Monks] than in other American men of the same age." They go on to say that diets "low in animal fats and associated with lowered serum cholesterol levels over a long period of years are not sufficient to prevent cardiovascular degeneration and high blood pressure."

The lesson we can draw from these studies is that fatty substances which become attached to the blood vessels certainly produce the condition we term arteriosclerosis or atherosclerosis. Of this there is no question. But viewing the evidence on man from Dachau, Korea, and elsewhere, and the evidence on wild vegetarian animals, there seems to be fairly conclusive proof that an extremely low-fat diet is no protection from cholesterol's forming in the body and being deposited on the artery walls—in the absence of some preventive factor.

What is that preventive factor, or factors? Could it be Vitamin E, in massive doses, perhaps, augmented by other substances? It is fairly apparent that animals in the wild, or in zoos, or the animal we call man does not have an optimum existence—else he would live much longer.

Dr. McKinney is continuing his study of the wild vegetarian animals. There are other studies which show that various apes, also noted vegetarians, suffer from cardiovascular diseases. Would additional Vitamin E solve their problem? We know that Vitamin E is effective on domestic animals and man; therefore, it should be on animals in the wild also.

Our doctors Shute, as well as other researchers, believe they have part of the clue to the puzzle of Vitamin E in relation to heart disease. Briefly, their thinking runs as follows: For the last sixty to seventy years, Vitamin E has been slowly but inexorably processed out of the American and British diets. For instance, present-day bread and flour, rice, corn, and the other cereal foods contain little Vitamin E. The Vitamin E which is available in fruits and vegetables is a poor source of alpha tocopherol, which is the only form of the vitamin which has been shown to be active in animals and in man. Also, as we mention elsewhere, the so-called "unsaturated" fatty oils derived from grains, such as corn, actually deplete the body of Vitamin E, even though, paradoxically, they contain fair amounts of the vitamin. (See page 118.)

Further, there is the problem of utilization. Meats such as steak and liver contain fair quantities of alpha tocopherol, but processing, storing, and cooking lower the Vitamin E content. It has been ascertained by researchers that Vitamin E, like Vitamin B12, is poorly utilized in the body, but this fact should not be alarming. In efficiency, the human body lies approximately between the electric motor (80 per cent efficient) and the steam engine (18 per cent), but considering the complexity of the work of the human body, this is a very high efficiency indeed. (We shall discuss utilization again in Chapter 8.)

Even under the most optimum conditions, supplementary amounts of the vitamin are recommended. Researchers, like Shute, P. L. Harris, and M. K. Horwitt, believe that the minimum set by the FDA is far too low, especially since both Harris and Horwitt, working independently, established that from 5 per cent to 7 per cent of adult Americans are actually notably deficient in Vitamin E. (See Bibliography.)

These tests compared persons having rapid destruction of

red blood cells with the normal, i.e., those persons whose stores of Vitamin E in the blood delayed for a standard period the destruction of red blood cells. According to these objective, *in vitro* tests, about 12,000,000 Americans are suffering from an outright deficiency of Vitamin E. There are undoubtedly many more millions of others who do not show an outright deficiency but are on the "borderline" in the so-called pre-clinical stage of deficiency. Remember, we are speaking of deficiencies, not of the amount of Vitamin E it takes to prevent and/or treat heart and circulatory disorders. The 12,000,000 figure is strangely reminiscent of the 12,000,000 heart disease sufferers in the U.S. We must emphasize that there have been no objective clinical tests of this correlation, but there should be.

Thus, the findings of our foremost Vitamin E researchers suggest that a good part of our mounting heart disease, particularly as it is manifested in America and other "civilized" countries, is due to the ever-increasing processing-out of the all-important Vitamin E which is essential to a healthy heart and circulatory system; heart troubles seem to have advanced in direct proportion to the decrease in Vitamin E (alpha tocopherol) in the contemporary diet. In 1896, at approximately the same time that Vitamin E and other vitamins were beginning to be processed out of bread and other cereal grains, an autopsy revealed the first identification of coronary thrombosis, one of the biggest killers among the myriad of troubles afflicting the heart today. (It was not until 1926 that coronary thrombosis was identified as the *actual* cause of death among persons who were previously considered normal and healthy.)

Very few researchers question the value of exercise, a well-balanced diet, and a fairly relaxed mental attitude. We have shown that cardiovascular disease is not caused by any single factor which can be applied to all societies, to all cultures, or to all individuals. Indeed, we have shown that all current hypotheses which plead "special causes" can be torn asunder. Yet no one would be so rash as to say that any one of the proposed hypotheses is absolutely invalid. For instance, should a deficiency of Vitamin E be recognized as the major factor in the increase of cardiovascular disease in recent years, it would still be necessary to exercise and eat properly and to avoid excessive weight and heavy stress.

There seems to be little doubt that one of the factors which plays a prominent role in the origin and treatment of most forms of heart disease is exercise—properly regulated, of course. Dr. Paul Dudley White, probably the best known heart specialist today because of his successful treatment of former President Eisenhower, is a vigorous proponent of exercise. His latest views were stated in an article in the *Atlantic Monthly* for October, 1963. (See below for some details.)

However, Dr. White is not alone. There is a rising tide of heart researchers who believe that properly governed exercise throughout life may help to prevent and/or control heart disease. There is much logic, reason, and scientific evidence to support this thesis. (See Bibliography: P. O. Astrand; W. W. Bauer; *Exercise and Fitness; Health and Fitness . . .*; W. F. Johnson; H. Kraus and W. Raab; and J. A. Faulkner.)

However, neither food (as eaten in the U.S., Great Britain, and other "civilized" countries) nor exercise seems to offer absolutely definitive answers to the riddle of heart disease. Heart disease is not an "old age" disease. We have more heart disease not because there are more people who are old but because it claims more and more victims in the middle-age and younger brackets. It is this rising proportion of deaths among the young and middle-aged persons which has so alarmed the authorities.

For instance, the aforementioned Dr. White began his *Atlantic* article with an account of a woman who was very disturbed about the probability of her sons, now eighteen and sixteen, dying of heart disease in their thirties. She cited the fact that "heart attacks" had killed the boys' great-grandfather at fifty-nine, their grandfather at fifty-one, and their father at forty-two. Each had died about a decade sooner than his father. Now, as we know, it is certainly "unscientific" to fear the sons' deaths in their thirties merely because death claimed the great-grand-father, grandfather, and father—each earlier than his father. Yet, who, trained or not in our scientific method, could resist wondering about the rather logical progression?

This correspondent's facts were not an isolated case of after-the-fact reasoning. Dr. White went on to cite an article in the *American Heart Journal* (July, 1963), by Dr. Samuel A. Levine (published in the *Atlantic Monthly* in July, 1963). Dr. Levine noted a study made of twenty fathers and twenty-one sons. He wrote: "The first evidence of coronary disease in the sons appeared at an age 13.1 years younger (48.1 years) than that of the fathers (61.2 years). The average age of death of eight sons was 54.8 years, and that of fourteen fathers was 68.7 years. . . . The evidence suggests that some factors are at work which cause coronary artery disease to appear at an earlier age and to run a more severe course in the present than in the previous generation." There are, of course, other studies such as the ones mentioned here which corroborate the fact that an increasingly larger number of young and middle-aged persons die suddenly from coronary and circulatory diseases.

Neither Dr. White nor Dr. Levine has much to offer to the prospective heart patient (particularly to Dr. White's worried correspondent). On exercise, Dr. White leans toward the gradual build-up program of exercising more and more each day whereas Dr. Levine relies less heavily on the exercise hypothesis. Both doctors suggest a good, healthy diet, some exercise, and a minimum of tension. Unfortunately, official scientific opinion is divided as to what constitutes a good, healthy diet for the heart, what proper exercise actually is, and how much worrying the human can take before it is significantly harmful.

In fact, as a contradistinction to the hope prospective heart patients are seeking, the erudite Dr. White quotes the writings of the ancient Roman, Pliny, the Elder, who, in his book on Natural History, wrote that "sudden deaths," which he called "life's supreme happiness" (non-violent, as differing from those occurring in wars, accidents, or murders), "are the most miraculous, and also frequent." Pliny notes that some of the various eminent Romans who died suddenly, from no obvious cause, "were so healthy and fit that they were thinking of going out for a walk."

All of the Romans mentioned by Pliny who died suddenly were well-born and wealthy; Dr. White thinks that luxurious living probably was a major factor in their mysterious deaths and that most probably the cause of death was from cardiovascular disease. He points out that almost every case of sudden death today—excluding violent actions—when autopsied, reveals significant degrees of coronary atherosclerosis.

If the thesis advanced by Dr. Shute and others holds true, i.e., that a Vitamin E deficiency is responsible for many coronaries or strokes, we can understand why the rich Romans did not enjoy good health: they ate too much, drank too much, exercised too little; very likely they did not eat the "plebian" coarse bread which was a major source of Vitamin E. We know with almost certainty that most heart disasters result from atherosclerosis or arteriosclerosis. This is true, whether our victim is a citizen of Imperial Rome, a modern American, Briton, or Russian, or whether it is a rat, gorilla, guinea pig, or chicken.

But the intriguing, vital question still plagues us: What are the origins, cures, and possible preventives? Alas, Dr. White (or any of his orthodox colleagues) can offer us nothing more definite than the following: ". . . from the evidence at hand, young people should avoid obesity, eat lightly of animal fats, work and exercise very hard throughout life." The fat admonition is hotly contested by even orthodox researchers, as we have previously noted.

All these various studies and theories on the cause of heart disease: lack of exercise, animal fats, stress, etc., are inconclusive and contradictory in light of the many studies on the subject. Let us then turn our attention to actual evidence on the efficacy of Vitamin E therapy in cases of cardiovascular disease in humans, and let us see whether we can come up with results that are conclusive and consistent.

We will not go into the dramatic details of each case. Rather, we would ask you to imagine the feelings, the emotions of each heart patient, regardless of whether he is helped in Canada, the Soviet Union, France, England, Italy, or many other countries from which the reports emanate.

One of the leading reports comes from Dr. V. R. O'Connor and Dr. J. P. S. Hodges of England. These doctors treated 350 patients for eight years for conditions ranging from general arteriosclerosis to congenital heart disease. Some of their patients were suffering from our old bug-a-boo coronary thrombosis; others were hit by angina, heart block, acute rheumatic fever, chronic rheumatic fever, and acute cerebral thrombosis. There are several other forms of cardiovascular diseases which these researcher-practitioners have treated with Vitamin E, but the aforementioned concern us the most here.

First, let us quote the conclusion of the British researchers: "Our final conclusion is that after 30 years' experience in both medicine and surgery, we believe that the alpha tocopherol treatment of cardiovascular and renal diseases, as suggested by Drs. E. V. and W. E. Shute, is one of the *greatest medical discoveries of the century.*" (Italics mine.) Remember these respected doctors spent more than thirty years treating heart ailments.

We shall next travel to Russia for confirmation which is there, too, in abundance. We will quote from the short abstract presented in the *Annotated Bibliography of Vitamin E* (published by the National Vitamin Foundation, 1958–1960). It was printed in a Soviet scientific journal (*Klin. Med.*), which one can obtain at the New York Academy of Medicine Library, 103rd Street and Fifth Avenue, New York City. The senior author, Dr. V. E. Anisimov, was studying a common form of heart ailment labeled "tachycardia," which is characterized by a rapid heart beat.

The medical team of Dr. Anisimov, *et al.,* was able to

obtain "clinical improvement" and "disappearance" of tachycardia attacks in twenty patients with arteriosclerosis and coronary sclerosis following the use of 50 I.U. of Vitamin E daily.[19]

In Austria, research was conducted at the Kaiser-Franz-
Josef-Spitals Hospital. There were three doctors working on the
study: H. Kern, O. Meissner, and R. Spies. (Their report,
published in a German heart journal, is listed in the Bibliography.) These doctors were primarily interested in the question: Could Vitamin E, in association with Vitamin A, alleviate
the symptoms of arteriosclerosis—the primary, acknowledged
precursor of heart failure? They studied 19 women and 16 men
whose ages ranged from 54 to 82 years. All had definite symptoms of arteriosclerosis. They were hospitalized for two weeks
so that they could be carefully tested for extraneous factors
other than the symptoms of arteriosclerosis.

After these tests were completed and the control group
established, the patients were given daily 210 international
units of Vitamin E and 90,000 units of Vitamin A. (In order
for the reader not to be confused at this point by the seemingly
high dosage of Vitamin A versus that of Vitamin E, let us state
that in a good serving of butter, liver, or many other foods,
you have the equivalent of 25,000 units of Vitamin A each
day. With Vitamin E, however, in which only alpha tocopherol
has proved to be effective, you probably receive only about
four to six units of alpha tocopherol daily.)

Of course, as Dr. Shute and others have discovered, a 210-
unit dosage of Vitamn E is rarely sufficient for preventing or
curing the symptoms of certain types of heart disease; nevertheless, such a dosage is sometimes effective if administered over
a long period of time. In this particular experiment in Vienna
the dosages were maintained for six months. The researchers
tell us that even on this small dosage, "improvement was apparent in six to eight weeks." The patients who were suffering
from the symptoms of arteriosclerotic disease reported relief

[19] See Bibliography for other corroborating Russian evidence: N. V.
Zhirnina and V. P. Stronkovskiy; J. J. Spirt, *et al.*

from their symptoms: headaches, insomnia, dizziness, and "ringing in the ears."

But more important from an objective viewpoint, in thirty of the high blood pressure victims, their pressure decreased by an average of 30 mm. (In layman's terms this means a considerable decrease.) Further, increased blood flow through the all-important arteries and veins was demonstrated by the oscillograph, the electronic machine which records the process. This writer has personally seen a fall in high blood pressure due to Vitamin E. A good friend of mine, to whom I recommended supplements of Vitamin E, reported after several weeks that her systolic pressure had dropped from 170 to 140. She does not dare tell her doctor for fear he will give her the same old story; *viz.,* that Vitamin E is no good for anything, otherwise, why wouldn't we see some articles in the AMA Journal about it? But my friend goes along quietly taking her Vitamin E—without having to resort to the usual pills for high blood pressure.

Let us now view some evidence from Paris, France, where, among numerous reports of Vitamin E activity in cardiovascular ailments, we examine the studies made by Dr. J. Loeper and Dr. P. Martin. (See Bibliography.) Drs. Loeper and Martin were experimenting with a derivative of Vitamin E called *alpha-tocopherol-quinone*. They were interested in lowering high blood pressure, which affliction, if unchecked, is a commonly recognized cause of "strokes" and "heart failure."

The French doctors selected forty patients whose high blood pressure (hypertension) had been long-standing and who had *not been helped by conventional methods* of treatment. They were, in medical terminology, "refractory" to the usual drugs employed to control hypertension.

The patients were treated with 150 to 300 I.U. daily for 3 to 8 weeks. The results: "A-Tocopherolquinone [*sic*] lowered blood pressure in 3 to 8 days"; and as they achieved over-all favorable response in 64 per cent of the patients, the doctors considered this figure "especially significant" because nothing else had been of *any* value.

They also set up a fairly high threshold of response since blood pressure *was* lowered to some degree in *all* patients, but the doctors in their statistics included only those favorable responses where pressure was dramatically lowered.

Dr. Loeper and Dr. Martin note that the most effective dose is 300 milligrams per day; when the treatment was stopped after 3 to 8 weeks, the blood pressure rose again "usually in 2 to 8 days, but sometimes, not for 2 or 3 weeks." The experimenters also observed that the treatment was well tolerated: "no allergic effects, no digestive or intestinal reactions, no sensation of fatigue, no capillary fragility or coagulation disturbances" (in contrast to the typical reactions that have been observed following conventional high blood pressure therapy).

In Stuttgart, Germany, we encounter the researches of Dr. E. Szirmai and Dr. G. Ruecker, who conducted their work at the Institute Erforsch, Blutgerinnung. There are scores of similar reports emanating from Germany, which has an almost unassailable reputation for preciseness and accuracy in scientific reports. Drs. Szirmai and Ruecker treated twenty-one patients who had arteriosclerotic disorders. They also had the means of checking scientifically the progress of their patients.

The patients were treated with Vitamin E (70 milligrams three times a day—a total of 210 mg.) and also with Vitamin B-6 (40 mg. per day), and Vitamin A (30,000 I.U.). The treatment lasted from four to six weeks, an unusually short time to prove the effects of any therapy. Yet sixteen of the patients exhibited both objective and subjective improvement; that is, machine and laboratory tests provided objective evidence and the patients themselves said that they felt better, were relieved of pain, etc. (subjective). Four other patients, according to the laboratory tests, showed improvement but claimed they did not—a fairly common phenomenon in medicine, when patients have a psychological block against getting well. Only *one* patient out of the twenty-one showed no improvement of any kind.

We shall now turn to Canada and report on a study made

by Dr. L. J. Clein, Dr. H. T. G. Williams, and Dr. R. A. Macbeth at the University of Alberta, Edmonton. Their report was published in the *Canadian Medical Association Journal* in 1962. These doctors were studying arterial disease occurring in the leg; all of their patients had what is known as "intermittent claudication." This disease is included in the present chapter because it is a vascular disease. The subjects under study suffered from a condition which makes it impossible for them to stand on their feet or walk for any length of time because the blood vessels in their legs were partially closed up by arteriosclerosis.

The study was a "double-blind" test, which means that unknown to them, half the patients received Vitamin E; the other half received "placebos," "pink pills" (sugar), which were of no worth, per se, in treating the disease. Of a group of twenty patients having a "poor distal bed"—i.e., the capillaries at the extremities of the legs were not functioning properly—all ten of the control group who were not given Vitamin E showed no change in their condition. In the Vitamin E-treated group, there were five successes, three classified as fair responses, and two failures. The doctors concluded that in patients with "distal bed occlusion, alpha tocopherol is a useful drug." From the sufferers' point of view, such relief from intermittent claudication with the help of Vitamin E therapy must have come as a welcome respite—and a study in understatement.

Let us now study a couple of patients recently seen at the Shute Institute in London, Ontario, Canada. The Drs. Evan and Wilfrid Shute have treated thousands of patients since their monumental discovery that Vitamin E was effective in cardiovascular disease, as well as other ailments. The Shutes have helped most of their patients, particularly when the patients were cooperative and followed through with their Vitamin E dosage after they left the Institute. Of course, human nature being what it is, it is difficult for some patients to believe that a "little pill" two or three times a day makes the difference between life or death for them. And, of course, it is doubly difficult to believe this fact when you are feeling "good."

In the June, 1963, *Summary,* the Shute Foundation's official journal, the two doctors reported on a random sampling of their cases.[20] A sixty-year-old man, listed in the Shute Clinic records as Case 430, was first seen at the clinic in April, 1948. He had had a coronary thrombosis attack the previous October. The patient, who was a horse trainer, complained of "lack of energy" and "occasional chest pains."

The electrocardiogram showed a "healed posterior scar," which, of course, was the aftermath of his previous coronary. Otherwise, no other abnormalities were found. The patient was put on a dosage of 360 I.U. of Vitamin E daily. This dosage seemed sufficient. As we have explained before, no one at that time knew that, in most cases, larger amounts of Vitamin E were necessary. (This factor has been the paramount bête-noire in most failures in experiments to date.[21]) For instance in 1948, Dr. Shute was probably the only researcher prescribing more than 300 I.U. daily. Nevertheless Case 430 got through the year training horses without suffering any chest pains until, in May, he developed slight "claudication"—no doubt the result of his extended walking and fairly heavy exercise.

He was advanced to 600 units of Vitamin E daily, but this dosage proved to be not enough for permanent relief, for two years later, in October, 1956, he suffered a recurrence. He was then advanced to 800 units. This dosage proved helpful, but in July of 1958 he had some difficulty in breathing (dyspnea). However, this condition did not last very long, and then *on his own,* he reduced the amount of Vitamin E slightly. He continued to improve, however, so that, by June of 1960, he was able to walk a half-mile before his left leg reacted with the gripping pains of claudication. He was smoking an occasional cigarette in spite of medical advice. Examination of both

[20] See Bibliography for other studies by Shute.
[21] See Appendix C.

legs revealed that the patient had both *arterial and venous* obstruction. This means he was (and probably had been) affected with arteriosclerotic obstruction in both phases of the circulatory systems. His dosage of alpha tocopherol was raised immediately back to 800 units.

This patient had continued to smoke an occasional cigarette throughout his treatment in spite of medical advice against it. As most persons know, in claudication tobacco is strictly proscribed since it constricts the blood vessels—an action which could be fatal to the already damaged or constricted vessels. In fact, there have been cases where the smoking of even one cigarette has brought on the horrible pains. Yet patient 430 did not give up smoking, which habit, as most readers probably know, is extremely hard to break.

In the winter of 1963, the patient suffered a mild *vasospasm;* that is, his blood vessels contracted and not enough blood could get through to nourish the cells properly. The only apparent result of this "attack" was that he could not speak for about an hour. However, he continued to take the 800 units of Vitamin E and seemed normal when he was examined again at the Shute Clinic in April, 1963. He possessed good exercise tolerance, so the report shows; he has had no recurrence of coronary thrombosis in fifteen years despite his history and his age; indeed, he has improved to the point where exercise does not bother him as it did many years ago before the start of Vitamin E. His claudication has been relieved enough so that today he leads a fairly normal life. This in spite of the fact that he has not followed the doctors' orders about smoking.

In retrospect, Dr. Shute comments that he would have treated Case 430 "with much larger doses fifteen years ago," but adds "he [the patient] has not done badly anyhow." Shute says that "in light of the recent vaso-spasm, we should carry him on at least 800 i.u. daily now." Not mentioning the sixteen-year-old coronary which has not recurred, Dr. Shute concludes: "A man who has both arterial and venous obstruction in his legs has a real problem, but alpha tocopherol is the best treatment for both, we feel."

Another case, a fifty-seven-year-old woman, No. 17219, was seen at the Shute Institute for the first time in April, 1962. This woman suffered the clutching pains of angina when she exerted herself. In addition she had ulcers of the small intestine (duodenal). Her electrocardiogram indicated evidence of coronary artery disease. This patient was started immediately on 600 units of alpha tocopherol. Within six months she had made a complete recovery, being free of all chest pain. She was now able to *swim a quarter of a mile!* When we reflect that so few "normal" individuals—and much younger than fifty-seven— can swim a quarter mile without being exhausted if not prostrated, we certainly have cogent proof of the wonder-working power of Vitamin E. However, No. 17219 still takes Vitamin E in order to prevent a return of the angina and also to obviate a coronary clot of which the angina patient must stand in continual fear.

Dr. Shute does not claim that Vitamin E will completely control *all* cases of angina. But it does greatly benefit in the majority of patients, particularly those whose condition is not so far advanced that their hearts need more oxygen and more blood than even Vitamin E can help supply.

Now, let us turn to the United States where Vitamin E is most neglected and is being bitterly fought by the cardiac specialists. This includes all of the organized medical groups and the various governmental agencies (which are under the domination of the organized medical groups).

Dr. Sol Hirsch of New York City, an internist of some repute, is among the courageous doctors who cannot be harmed by the organized groups. He has reached a stage in life where, because of his undisputed, long record (46 years) of successful treatment of thousands of patients, he does not have to worry about his reputation or about acquiring new patients. Among other accomplishments, he has developed a highly successful, original method of treating migraine headaches and has delivered lectures before various medical societies. He has also published in various medical journals, including the *New York State Journal of Medicine*.

During the last ten years, Dr. Hirsch has treated many heart disease patients, and reports with confidence on his "very successful treatment of heart and related cardiovascular conditions with Vitamin E." He believes, as do many nutritionists, that Vitamin E therapy is enhanced by the addition of multivitamins and other supplements. These include the B-complex, Vitamin C with bioflavonoids, dried liver tablets, calcium, and wheat germ oil concentrate. He is an advocate of the theory that vitamins work best in conjunction with each other and should never be taken alone because they may upset the metabolic balance or dynamic equilibrium of the body—even if they are shown to be non-toxic in huge quantities if taken singly. (Actually the only vitamins that have been proven to be toxic are Vitamins A and D and possibly elements of the B-complex, and yet even these have to be administered for considerable periods of time in tremendous dosages—usually without the counteracting effect of other vitamins—before any evidence of toxic effects are noted.)

Dr. Hirsch is his own best example of Vitamin E therapy. Like so many doctors, he is constantly overworked. And like so many other doctors, he developed a heart condition some years ago. It was a myocardiac insufficiency, sometimes known as coronary insufficiency, which occurs as a result of the heart's decreased function as a pump: it cannot force enough blood through the arteries to operate efficiently; therefore, the tissues and cells, deprived of sufficient oxygen and other nutrients, send an urgent message to the brain for more oxygen. The overstrained heart usually cannot respond, but the lungs can. Result: fast breathing in a desperate attempt to convey more oxygen to the cells and to the heart itself—which is caught in a vicious cycle of not being able to function properly because of lack of nutrients; naturally, the longer this process goes on, the more inadequate is the heart's response. Then frequently comes the dreaded angina attack with its horrible pains.

The heart sends out its own urgent appeal to the brain for more oxygen. The brain responds by redistributing available blood resources, with priority to the heart, for without heart function for more than four to seven minutes, there would be no existence. Wherewith the victim of the coronary (or the coronary insufficiency) will lie down as the blood drains down from the brain. If the brain sends the blood down too fast, thereby shutting itself off too quickly, the victim will experience a fainting spell, for now only the hypothalamus—the old, middle brain—is working. The thinking areas have gone into seclusion pending more fuel. Or perhaps enough blood has remained in the cerebrum (the consciously thinking part of the brain) to maintain consciousness. In some instances it would have been better if the patient had lost consciousness, for, as we have described in another chapter, the fear of death may send the thinking part of the brain into absolute panic and thereby disrupt the automatic machinery of the body which could have saved the victim.

The reader can readily see how complex and dangerous such a condition can be. For the doctor who has had such a personal experience, the treatment and prevention of such an attack become doubly meaningful. When I saw Dr. Hirsch (November, 1963), he looked much younger than his actual age. He told me that he had been taking Vitamin E for the last several years, along with the vitamins and food supplements, and that the treatment was controlling his heart condition very well. *Surprisingly well,* I might add, since I know Dr. Hirsch as a friend and I am aware that he almost never rests in spite of his age and his advice to his patients—but what doctor does?

Out of the hundreds of patients Dr. Hirsch has treated with Vitamin E to their great benefit, let us mention one at random. This patient, who came to Dr. Hirsch about ten years ago, had a myocardiac condition with a valvular block. He was taking digitalis with very little effect. Dr. Hirsch instituted Vitamin E along with the other supplements. This man had been desperate, for he was heaving and puffing on the slightest exertion. Within one month, however, he had discarded his digitalis and was living in excellent health, performing his duties without difficulty. He continued the therapy for ten years, during which time he had no further trouble with his heart.

Dr. Hirsch has other patients, of course, some as dramatic, others not so dramatic, but almost all nevertheless proving the worth of Vitamin E. This doctor is one of the few in the United States who has dared to challenge the verdict of the orthodox.

Dr. Hirsch supports what we have been reiterating throughout this book. The evidence concerning any new therapy is automatically rejected under our present system if it is not under the aegis of orthodox and, therefore, official patronage or supervision. In medicine, almost all monumental discoveries have, for the most part, *one* man's name attached to them, or possibly two who work in extremely close cooperation such as Banting and Best, the discoverers of insulin. And, of course, we know that penicillin was not discovered by a team but by Sir Alexander Fleming, who was recently quoted by the Denver *Post,* among others, as having said: "Penicillin sat on the shelf for twelve years while I was called a quack. I can only think of the thousands who died needlessly because my peers would not use my discovery."

6

Vitamin E in Other Conditions

How many times have you heard or read that, because you live in the United States, you are living in the healthiest country in the world? How many times have you been told that U.S. medicine is par excellence, so high it cannot be compared with that of other countries?

Irreverent question: how many major advances in medicine had their origins in the U.S.? You can count on the fingers of one hand the truly significant discoveries which really originated between our northern-most latitude and the Mexican border. Indeed, the discovery of ether anesthesia was just such a monumental finding; this discovery was made almost simultaneously by William Morton and Crawford W. Long working independently, and both can attribute their finds to serendipity —that stumbling on something fortunate without expecting it. At that time, there were no vast teams of researchers and no authoritarian bureaucrats to tell anyone what to work on, how he should do it, and when and, also, how he should publish his findings (if any).

So often important medical discoveries are announced in the United States, yet we find that the basis of the "discovery" originated in another country. For instance, the world credits Walter Reed with the discovery that a certain type of female mosquito causes Yellow Fever. Yet a careful study of the record reveals that Dr. Reed acknowledges his indebtedness to an old Scotch-Cuban physician, Carlos Findlay, for the hypothesis, accompanied by some proof, that mosquitoes were responsible for the (then) deadly Yellow Jack. (I have investigated the actual events pertaining to the cause and solution of Yellow Fever, with the invaluable aid of a medical volunteer, Gust Lambert, who was close to Reed and other doctors involved in this, the first, really controlled experiment on human beings; one day, we shall relate this story, which version differs considerably from the official account.)

The same could be said of effective vaccines, antibiotics, "tranquilizers," and electronic devices such as ultra-sound and the electroencephalograph. The reason? American medicine is caught in an official medical strait-jacket.

Certainly, the work of medical teams in the United States is essential and international corroboration is invaluable. But the important point is that money, as it is usually allocated by both governmental and private sources, somehow does not seem to produce the desired results because it is often controlled by medical politicians both in government and out. The ambition of these men is to make, maintain, and perpetuate the legend that the more money spent for research, the more results will be forthcoming.

Yet, of the over 183,000,000 inhabitants of the "healthiest nation in the world," 74,000,000 have one or more chronic conditions. These figures emanate from one of the same official agencies[22] which blithely assure us that we are, indeed, the healthiest nation on earth, the United States Public Health Service. And, of course, such propaganda is "corroborated" by the FDA and the AMA which have developed a case of model schizophrenia: on the one hand, we are the healthiest nation on earth having the best food and the best medical research; on the other hand, we have the sorry facts and figures. One-fourth of our school children cannot pass an elementary examination in physical fitness which European school children and Soviet Union children laugh about because it's so easy. About one-half of our draftees called for service are not accepted, for physical or mental reasons, and the standards for these exams

[22] See "Current Estimates . . ."; also "Health Statistics. . . ."

are not very high. If a recruit has some "minor" condition such as a hernia or bad teeth, it will not render him ineligible—especially in war time; the government is concerned only with "real" problems such as heart disease, cancer, and insanity.

In a recent special report on chronic conditions issued by the Public Health Service, 74,000,000 sufferers in the United States were counted. You may say, these must represent the older segment of our society since we're living so much longer nowadays. Wrong on both premises. First, at the time the report was released (1963), there were only 17 million persons over sixty-five. As for the premise which is being disseminated throughout the country, that we are living longer, alas, this also is a fiction.

The Metropolitan Life Insurance Company's report on comparative longevity, along with other studies, disproves the myth that you or I will live much longer than our fathers or grandfathers—once we have escaped the childhood diseases (which now are largely eliminated by antibiotics and other drugs). There are more oldsters around and there will be still more because more of us have escaped these once devastating childhood diseases. And, of course, fewer die of infectious diseases such as tuberculosis, pneumonia, or malaria which have largely been conquered by drugs. This fact does not mean, however, that the average man is living appreciably longer—it merely means that *more people* are living longer and, therefore, have a chance to exist until 70—or if their stamina is above average, they may live far beyond that. However, the percentage of adult persons who manage to escape death until 70 has not changed appreciably in the last fifty years. Since there are more so-called "senior citizens," the statistics have been widely misinterpreted to "prove" that man's life expectancy beyond the age of 30 has been noticeably increased. There is no reason, however, why man's real life expectancy should not be increased. But the fact that to date it has not, provides us with a major reason why the insurance companies are able to erect enormous buildings and spend millions of dollars in advertising. (Since the above was written, even more undeniable corroboration has been presented in a report by the U.S. Public Health Service. Entitled, "The Change in Mortality Trend in the United States" (1964), the study admits that the American death rate has not improved in the last decade. The report suggests that our failure to make progress against chronic and degenerative diseases [and thereby boosting the death rate] and that our failure to "become healthier" during the last ten years may be due to "radio-active fallout, air pollution, and other man-made hazards." Many would disagree with this interpretation; nevertheless, the fact remains that we are not living longer percentage-wise. Denmark, Norway, Sweden, Japan, and the Netherlands are among the many countries which have a lower death rate than the U.S.)

But let us return to the appalling report of chronic conditions issued by the Public Health Service. Of the 74 million chronically ill, 19 million have their activities limited or impaired, 4 million are so seriously ill they cannot function in usual activities such as working or keeping house. Heart disease, of course, is our big leader in this group, accounting for 24 per cent of the total. Arthritis and rheumatism follow with 16 per cent; and visual impairment next with 11 per cent.

You may be wondering about all this talk about chronic conditions and what it has to do with Vitamin E. Well, as a rather conservative estimate, about half those chronic sufferers could be helped by Vitamin E, and very likely more than half of the diseases could have been prevented or controlled by Vitamin E.

We know, for instance, that cardiovascular diseases alone account for more than half the deaths in the United States. In 1962, there were 1,757,000 deaths from various causes. Diseases of the cardiovascular system accounted for the staggering total of 954,870. The percentage, as we have explained previously, is mounting steadily. 1964 will see the total explode well over the 1,000,000 mark. (In sharp contrast, cancer deaths accounted for only 277,110 in 1962. Cancer is the number two killer.)

Now arthritis and rheumatism which afflict at least 11 to 12 million persons are not killers, and they are almost never categorized as the cause of death; they are the cripplers, the incapacitators. However, victims often wish they were dead, their pains are so agonizing.

As for the remainder of the chronic maladies, such as diabetes, polio, muscular dystrophy, multiple sclerosis, and epilepsy, the public is constantly being bombarded with calls to contribute to research; yet the number of persons dying from these afflictions is so small that statisticians hardly bother with them. Of course, to a person suffering from muscular dystrophy, such a disease is the most important ailment in the world; his friends and relatives believe so too; it is most distressing to witness the gradual wasting away of a person's body when you know there is nothing to be done about it except to support future medical research. This futility is based on the assumption that all avenues of therapy have been thoroughly explored and that nothing more can be done for the patient. Yet, with muscular dystrophy patients, reports from all over the world present some scientific evidence that at least one-fifth to one-half of such sufferers, who are treated with massive doses of Vitamin E, are helped—in some cases, dramatically so. If research funds were available for the study of Vitamin E in relation to muscular dystrophy, multiple sclerosis, and other such relatively rare diseases, we would no doubt hear a different story from the one we are continually forced to hear: "At present, there is no hope except in the dollars you contribute."

Unfortunately, however, almost none of the dollars you contribute to fund-raising organizations find their way into a serious, prolonged study of Vitamin E—this fact applies to heart disease as well as to the less prevalent ailments. If researchers in Vitamin E had only an infinitesimal portion of the millions which Congress and the private collection groups, such as the American Heart Association, allocate to studies of the heart, there would be a marked decrease in fatalities from cardiovascular diseases and relief for many other conditions as well. Let us now examine briefly some of the diseases and afflictions other than those of the cardiovascular system which Vitamin E has proved useful in relieving or controlling.

WOUNDS AND BURNS

Now while wounds and burns are not listed under the category of chronic diseases, nevertheless, they constitute a significant form of disablement. Wounds and injuries received while in the armed services afflict millions, as do the burns and injuries incurred in everyday civilian life. Vitamin E, when used as an ingredient in an ointment at the site of the wound or burn, and also taken internally, has been found by no less than seven researchers in various countries (see Appendix A, p. 151), to hasten the healing of the wound or burn—and most significantly—to reduce the amount of scar tissue in some cases. The vitamin seems to soften and dissolve the tissues which form a scar. (The ointment can be obtained without a prescription in most stores wherever vitamins are sold.) Of course, the Shutes were in the forefront of this work and have verified the various foreign reports with many photographs of their own "before and after" patients treated with Vitamin E who had been wounded, burned, or had gangrenous limbs.

Dr. Evan Shute considers this faculty of Vitamin E to be one of the most important discoveries that he and his brother have made in the long list of beneficent effects attributed to the vitamin. For instance, since burns are the primary consequences of an atomic or nuclear attack (among those surviving the initial blast), Vitamin E could be the means of saving thousands of persons from disfiguration. The vitamin has been shown to lessen the effects of radiation burns as well as burns caused by "ordinary" means. There is no other inexpensive, effective, safe, and self-applicable therapy yet developed for radiation burns—or for that matter, burns of *any* nature.

As soon as he had irrefutable proof of Vitamin E's action on wounds and burns, Dr. Evan Shute wrote to the defense departments of the United States, England, and Canada, presenting the aforementioned scientific observations. Readers of this book do not have to be crystal-ball gazers to know what happened. The officials referred the matter to their medical advisors. The advisors being "sound" and "orthodox," naturally believed that Vitamin E was worthless in any therapeutic capacity—further, that Shute was a "bug" on Vitamin E and had "lost his scientific perspective."

Result: You do not see Vitamin E tablets or ointment in any Civilian Defense Recommendation for Survival, nor do you see them in any soldier's kit. Well, while we hope fervidly that total war never occurs, we do also hope with equal fervor that readers of this book will obtain both Vitamin E tablets and ointment. They may be put to good use, not only in war, but now, as an ointment on burns, wounds, indolent ulcers, and many other skin conditions.

DIABETES

In popular belief, this disease has been long "conquered" by the use of insulin and an adjusted diet. This concept, however, is far from accurate. It is true that insulin, in conjunction with a rigidly regulated diet, can control the obvious manifestations of high blood sugar; but what is not generally known, except to an ever-increasing group of diabetic specialists, is that even with the best insulin supervision and dietary controls, 85 per cent of all diabetics on long-term treatment (15 years) develop other complicating diseases such as coronaries, cataracts, leg gangrene, and ulcers. Dr. E. P. Joslin, co-author of *The Treatment of Diabetes Mellitus,* noted that as treatment with insulin progressed, so did deaths from vascular causes among insulin-treated patients. For instance, between 1898–1914—before insulin—the death rate from vascular diseases among diabetics was only 17.5 per cent as compared with the period 1944–1948 when the vascular death rate of diabetics increased to 66.6 per cent! (See Bibliography for Joslin's work.)

Foreign statistics give even more impressive evidence that diabetics (all insulin-treated) become victims of other diseases, especially those in the cardiovascular realm. Among the researchers corroborating Joslin, *et al.,* were Drs. Travia and Scapelato, who, working independently, found that diabetics suffered from various forms of cardiovascular diseases. The percentage ranged from 80–90 per cent. (See Bibliography.)

But it was Dr. Ugo Butturini, of Bologna, Italy, who probably made the most monumental findings concerning Vitamin E in relation to diabetic heart disease. Dr. Butturini and associates studied 129 diabetic patients with practically all forms of cardiovascular disturbances. They not only discovered that Vitamin E, given in adequate doses (average 300 I.U.), was beneficial in most forms of cardiovascular diseases in diabetics, but that it also eliminated entirely the need for insulin in 50 per cent of the patients, reduced the need in 30 per cent; was ineffective in only 20 per cent. Dr. Butturini's classic contributions are recorded in the extensive list in the Bibliography.

Almost no diabetics today die of diabetes per se, but the disease produces a steady degeneration in the circulatory system which leads to many "complications" of diabetes, for which insulin has no discernible value. It should be emphasized, however, that before the discovery of insulin by Banting and Best, the outcome of diabetes was invariably fatal—usually five to six years at the maximum after the initial diagnosis.

Medical men since then have reasoned that diabetes was far more complicated than the failure of the pancreas to produce enough insulin to control the sugar in the blood stream. The disease also struck other areas of the body which had little or nothing to do with the insulin-sugar balance, notably the circulatory system. This attack was particularly evident in the tiny capillaries and in the smaller blood vessels which have the titanic task of supplying the individual cells with the elements essential for an effective metabolism; somehow, this function of the capillaries was being disturbed. For one thing, the permeability of the capillaries was altered: that is, their walls were no longer responsive in this normal fashion. The nutrient substances carried by the blood were leaking out the capillary walls and not penetrating the tissue cells; also, waste products of the cells could not gain their accustomed entrance to the blood cells by "reverse" penetration, thence to be transported back to the various organs for elimination or to be changed into neutral, harmless substances. Therefore, deprived of nutrients and unable to rid themselves of harmful materials, the cells died.

Now, as we know, the death of one cell makes small difference to the body since we have an astronomical number. New cells are constantly replacing those which die every second we live, but when millions of cells start dying in the same place it becomes a serious matter.

Such is roughly what happens in gangrene, leg ulcers, Buerger's Disease, or "intermittent claudication." This is why diabetics so frequently are afflicted with, not only these aforementioned diseases, but many others as well. Diabetics have a circulation problem which is clearly evidenced by their not dying from diabetes but from diseases which once were considered totally unrelated to diabetes.

Dr. Joslin deplored the attitude of most authorities that diabetes could be written off as "conquered" by insulin alone. In fact Dr. Joslin went so far as to state that insulin masked the real culprits in diabetes and that it comforted the diabetic into thinking he was well for a time; yet all the while he was developing and dying from complications produced by arteriosclerosis.

Now because of Vitamin E's qualities as an oxygen conserver, vasodilator, regulator of the cells' permeability, and muscle stimulant, among other qualities, it should be able to assist the body in managing diabetes. There is another attribute which several researchers found: It actually decreases the blood stream sugar in a number of patients, just as it decreases high blood pressure in a number of hypertensives. Its whole operation in the body, as we have previously mentioned, is toward the normal, toward maintaining *homeostasis,* the tendency of the body toward the normal.

The Shutes, along with the previously mentioned Dr. Butturini, were among the first researchers to discover Vitamin E's role in treating diabetes. They have now treated hundreds of diabetics with partial to completely successful results in most of their cases—provided that damage has not been done that is irreversible. They also have found that a diabetic who is given large doses of Vitamin E can oftentimes dispense with insulin altogether. In most cases, insulin can be eliminated entirely (usually with the early victims) or else cut to a fraction of the former dose. In 80 per cent of all diabetics, need for insulin can be either eliminated or drastically reduced. The Shutes admit to failure in 20 per cent of the cases, but as we have seen, pathological, irreversible changes of the organs and tissues frequently make 100 per cent success impossible.

The Shutes are backed up in their findings on diabetes by no less than thirty-five studies all over the world, and all, of course, performed by reputable researchers who have published in leading foreign medical journals.[23] Sadly enough, most of these favorable reports on Vitamin E are kept from you but, even more sadly, are kept from your doctor as well.

DISEASES OF PREMATURES AND INFANTS

Since cow's milk is, for humans, deficient in Vitamin E, Vitamins A and C, nicotinic acid, linoleic acid, fat and iron, it is necessary that these substances be added to the infant's formula. In reviewing these findings, Dr. F. C. Aitken of the Rowett Research Institute, Aberdeen, Scotland, and Dr. F. E. Hytten, of the University of Aberdeen, recommended Vitamin E supplementation in order to prevent destruction of infants' red blood cells. Unfortunately, Vitamin E and the others are almost never added, because of the current medical faddism about extra vitamins being unnecessary, either for the pregnant mother or the new-born or the premature, or the child or the adult, or the aging individual.

It has been shown in scores of reports that premature infants and even so-called "normal" new-borns are deficient in

[23] See Bibliography: Haimovici; Nelson.

Vitamin E. For instance, the mother has about twelve times more Vitamin E in her blood than her new-born child. The reason postulated for this is that Vitamin E, being oil soluble instead of water soluble, does not cross the placental barrier as easily as do most nutrients (such as the B-complex vitamins which are water-soluble and, therefore, blood-soluble). It takes massive amounts of Vitamin E in the blood of the mother for it to be evidenced in the foetus or the new-born. The mother's milk, however, does contain enough Vitamin E to build up the new-born child's reserves of alpha tocopherol in about seven weeks, while infants fed "formula" diets do not achieve corresponding levels of Vitamin E for two years. These findings were reported by Dr. H. H. Gordon, *et al.*, among others. (See Bibliography.) Yet today, most infants are deprived of breast-feeding, and their cow's milk formula rarely is supplemented with Vitamin E or many of the other known essentials in which cow's milk is deficient.[24]

It is a noteworthy observation that in most common ailments of premature and full-term infants, there is a serious depletion of Vitamin E. Even more significant is the fact that when these infants are given Vitamin E, in most cases, the diseases clear up. One of the leading workers in pediatrics who discovered these startling facts is Dr. F. Gerloczy of the University Medical School, Budapest. Dr. Gerloczy has conducted many series of tests on prematures, the new-born, and young children. In all of the disease conditions studied, which ranged from scleroderma (a watery swelling, usually following an acute infection which is frequently fatal to infants) to growth retardation in young children, the researcher found Vitamin E deficiency in direct proportion to the severity of the condition. Placed on Vitamin E therapy, the conditions were usually eliminated or well-controlled. (See Wenig and Westphal.)

As an example, let us take Dr. Gerloczy's classic study of 320 prematures afflicted with scleroderma. Mortality had been

[24] See Bibliography: R. Beckman; L. S. Baur; H. M. Nitowsky, *et al.*; N. S. Scrimshaw, *et al.*; E. V. Shute; W. A. Blanc.

about 75 per cent. With Vitamin E therapy, the mortality dropped to 27 per cent. Dr. Gerloczy also noted Vitamin E's diuretic effect which took the excess water out of the infant's body quickly and safely. (See Bibliography, "The Importance of Vitamin E in Pediatrics," *Orvosi Hetilap.*)

Other researchers throughout the world have corroborated Dr. Gerloczy's findings. Drs. H. H. Gordon, H. M. Nitowsky, J. T. Tildon, and S. Levin, working jointly at Sinai Hospital and Johns Hopkins School of Medicine found that Vitamin E therapy greatly benefits infants and children with diseases of the pancreas and gall bladder. Dr. R. Beckman, of the University of Freiburg, Germany, found that Vitamin E is particularly beneficial in diseases of the liver. He also found that a dose of 300 milligrams of Vitamin E given to women at the start of delivery reduces the incidence of brain hemorrhages in the child. He recommends large doses of Vitamin E for slow-growing children. (More confirmation can be found in the references in the Bibliography.) All these researchers recommend supplemental doses of Vitamin E for infants, particularly those not breast-fed.

STERILITY

According to all medical data, about 10 per cent of U.S. marriages are sterile. Even more connubial unions produce afflicted offspring or else the wife cannot carry the foetus for nine months. A miscarriage ensues, which naturally disturbs both the husband and wife. It is worse still if the progeny turns out to be mentally retarded, or a Mongolian idiot, or arrives in the form of what the medical profession calls a "monster." This latter term applies to queer physical anomalies. We need not go into details here, but the reader, should he be interested in the subject matter, is herewith referred to a classic book in its field, written by two doctors, George M. Gould and Walter L. Pyle, *Anomalies and Curiosities of Medicine,* recently reissued by Julian Press. There are more such anomalies than most people would imagine. Often these unfortunate ones are carefully hidden from their parents' sight and public observation by being placed in institutions.

Is there a way to prevent, not only the anomalies, but the miscarriages, and to provide otherwise childless couples with a normal baby? The orthodox will tell you that the chances are very slim, but that they are "on the track of this problem."

Recently, a medical report stated that the husband's sperm fluid may produce an allergic reaction in the wife which prevents conception. This process, according to the authors, Drs. Robert R. Franklin and C. Dean Dukes of Baylor University College of Medicine, is somewhat similar to an antigen—or a foreign protein—being injected into the body after the body has prepared defenses against a specific foreign protein.

Official American medicine will go to any lengths to prove anything it wishes, but is it not most astounding that it did not choose to validate the already existing European and Canadian studies concerning sterility in the human? The European studies are so conclusive as to the value of Vitamin E in sterility that it is almost impossible to believe that they were not followed up in this country. This observation does not reflect on the validity of the "allergic" findings developed in this country. It merely means that for many years we have had one of the prime keys to sterility, regardless of allergic responses, and have chosen to ignore it.

There are approximately fifty well-controlled studies which demonstrate the value of Vitamin E in producing healthy offspring in previously barren couples.[25] There are also hundreds of animal studies which corroborate this observation in practically all mammalian species.[26] If the reader remembers the classic experiments of the Darlington-Chassels study of race horses, with regard to increasing the production of thoroughbreds, then he may anticipate that the same results apply in all mammals, including man. This property of Vitamin E—that of

[25] See Bibliography: R. Bayer; E. Lindner; E. V. Shute; Da Rugna; Horne.
[26] See Chapter 4.

improving the quality of the sperm as well as the general health of both parents—has been noted throughout the history of the vitamin. In fact, as we have mentioned previously, this ability to induce the production of healthy offspring caused it to be tagged an "anti-sterility vitamin," and this is still considered by many medical authorities to be the vitamin's prime function.

It has also been indicated that there is a high degree of correlation between "habitual abortion," whether caused by defective sperm or ova or other factors, and congenital defects in the infant. For instance, a woman who suffers frequent miscarriages is more apt to give birth to an abnormal child than a woman who does not abort. Also, those who produce an abnormal baby are more likely to repeat the same sad experience than couples who have healthy offspring. Therefore, any agent, such as Vitamin E, which would reduce sterility would *necessarily* tend to obviate the miscarriages as well as the "anomalies."

Throughout our extensive research on Vitamin E the phrase frequently appears, "There were *no* anomalies with Vitamin E therapy, whereas there were the usual ones before." Any agent which can cure abnormal conditions or diseases produced by deficiencies can also *prevent* them. Witness the action of Vitamin C in the prevention as well as the cure of scurvy; likewise Vitamin B-12 and pernicious anemia; niacin and pellagra; B-1 and beriberi; Vitamin D and rickets; and so on.

Fully a dozen experiments demonstrate that the male of the species is partially to blame for infertility and, therefore, he is very likely partly responsible for the production of anomalies and miscarriages.

Now, can the sperm be qualitatively improved so that they can mate with the ova and produce healthy offspring? The answer, of course, is yes. Both male and female should take a course of Vitamin E therapy at least one to three months before attempted conception, and then, after conception, should continue with Vitamin E—particularly the woman, if she wants to carry her offspring for the nine months without too much trouble. After conception the husband may abandon Vitamin E except that he, as are all others, may be a good candidate for a heart condition if he does not continue with Vitamin E. However, for our purposes here, we will ignore the father after conception because his role is then finished as the producer of a healthy child.

Out of the scores of studies reporting the capability of Vitamin E to aid in the problem of sterility we have selected a typical example for presentation here.

One such study comes from West Germany, conducted by Dr. R. Bayer (see Bibliography). Dr. Bayer treated 100 married couples. More than half of the group were victims of "primary infertility": Although the couples were able to conceive, they lost 100 per cent of their conceptions. These couples had 144 pregnancies and had lost all of them prior to Vitamin E treatment. Yet there were seventy-nine pregnancies after pre-conception treatment with Vitamin E, and only two women lost their babies, whereas *all* women had aborted *all* their babies before Vitamin E therapy. Dr. Bayer was, thus, able to reduce failure from 100 per cent to 2½ per cent.

Dr. Bayer's second group, those with "secondary infertility" (the couples had some successful births rather than total failure) had been able to achieve a total of only 38 births out of 101 pregnancies. Yet with his standard dosage of 100 milligrams daily for one month for the husband and 200 milligrams daily for three months prior to conception for the wife, Dr. Bayer observed *100 per cent* favorable results. In other words, from forty-one pregnancies in the second group, there were forty-one births, all of them healthy offspring.

But Dr. Bayer, being a disciplined, fearless scientist, of a calibre of which, sad to say, we have so few in this country, carried his experiment even further. He wanted to prove it was Vitamin E and Vitamin E alone which produced the abrupt change in sterility. In *both* groups, he lowered the Vitamin E intake to one-third of its former intake. Result: when the husbands in the first group ("primary sterility") were lowered to one-third of their former intake of Vitamin E, the loss of babies, which was formerly 100 per cent, was reduced to only 33 per cent (thirty-one pregnancies this time), instead of 2½ per cent when the heavier dosage was taken. In the second group ("secondary infertility"), when the amount of Vitamin E was reduced to one-third of the former amount, the loss of babies was reduced from 61 per cent (without Vitamin E) to 21 per cent, instead of 100 per cent successful births as with the heavy dosage. Thus, we see that Dr. Bayer and his associates have not only proved that Vitamin E can be essential in human sterility and the health of the offspring but that the actual dosage of the vitamin must be therapeutic in order to achieve optimum results, i.e., a successful conception and a successful birth. Dr. Bayer's studies—particularly those concerned with sperm improvement—have been corroborated in many other experiments throughout the world, though none was probably as definitive. (See Bibliography: Zanatu, Horne, Nickolowski.)

It is most interesting to note that in not one of the experiments where the man and wife were under intensive Vitamin E therapy has there ever been recorded the birth of a monster or even a mentally retarded child. There were hundreds of men, women, and children involved in these experiments and, by all laws of percentages, there should have been several monsters, and quite a few mentally retarded children. Therefore, Vitamin E, in playing its many beneficial roles within the body, is able to improve the quality of the sperm in the human male; and, judging from the mass of evidence, both animal and human, Vitamin E is able to alter the female's reception of the sperm and later to provide a good environment for the developing foetus. In addition, Vitamin E can cross the vital placental wall—although with some difficulty[27]—whence the foetus receives the necessary nutrients from its mother—nutrients essential to its growth and well-being. It is apparent that large

---

[27] There are hundreds of animal studies which demonstrate beyond any question the fact that the life-conserving qualities of Vitamin E are transmitted to the foetus.

amounts of Vitamin E given to the mother can, in turn, assist the rapidly-growing organism which, within a remarkably short time, becomes the air-breathing mammalian we know as a human baby.

There are thousands of animal studies to corroborate the fact that almost all mammalians need much Vitamin E and, when deprived of it, the organism will suffer injury to almost every cell in its body. Therefore, this deprivation of Vitamin E tends toward fostering diseases of every sort imaginable. Is it not reasonable to suppose that since every cell in the body is affected by the abundance of Vitamin E—or its lack—almost every disease known to man or beast is similarly affected?

Now, as we have stated, Dr. Bayer's essential findings have been corroborated by many researchers throughout the world, working with animals, largely, and later with humans: that Vitamin E therapy previous to conception does, indeed, enhance the chances of a successful pregnancy.

Many researchers have shown that Vitamin E therapy (oftentimes in conjunction with B-complex and other supplements) prevents the birth of monsters or congenitally deformed babies. There is an overwhelming amount of evidence in animal experiments to support this work which has been done on human beings. Again, the same rules by which Vitamin E operates in the human or the animal, hold true in the human or the animal embryo.

Now I shall inject a personal note: I have a good friend, Anna G. Morin of Framingham, Massachusetts who provides us with an excellent and typical case history of what Vitamin E can do for couples who wish babies but cannot have them. Mrs. Morin had her first child after a most difficult delivery. Then she went through a horrible period of three miscarriages until she heard about Vitamin E and wrote Dr. Shute for advice. While we cannot reprint her correspondence with Dr. Shute because of lack of space, we can observe that this great man spent a great deal of time with her and her husband advising them on Vitamin E for a successful pregnancy.

Both husband and wife were started on Vitamin E. Result:

the next pregnancy was a success. So was their next one! And judging by the letters which Dr. Shute has written them, he appears to be as happy as they are, which again proves this doctor is as much a humanitarian as a researcher.

STRESS AND OLD AGE

One of the most discussed men in science today is Hans Selye, Ph.D., at the University of Montreal. His experiments[28] with animals placed under stress have all tended to demonstrate that stress (tension) is, at the least, responsible for inducing the conditions which lead to most illnesses. Now stress can be produced experimentally in laboratory animals in a variety of ways; for instance, it can be "physical," such as having rats swim in ice water and comparing their survival time, or it can be a "mental frustration," such as giving an animal a problem too difficult for it to solve in order to reach food. Since rats are somewhat close to man in a nutritional sense—and since most illness, in the broader view, are nutritional in origin—the experiments have a great validity for the human being.

Dr. Selye's most recent research has a particular interest for readers of this book. He, together with his associates, M. Cantin and Jean-Marie Dieudonne, have succeeded in reproducing the signs and symptoms of "old age" in the young rat. They take litter mates for "controls" to prove that their aging process is valid; in other words, rats from the same litter can be made "old," and they die in a matter of weeks while their brothers and sisters who are not subjected to the treatment, live out a normal life. Selye is attempting to learn the exact process that explains why and how we grow old. Once this process is discovered, there may be ways and means to combat it, hold it off, or even reverse it.

His recent studies afford many valuable clues to the aging process. It is rather an amazing fact to those uninitiated in the seeming conspiracy against Vitamin E that although Selye's studies were published in the *Journal of Experimental Medicine*

[28] See Cantin, *et al.*

and Surgery, in 1962, the reports in the various other medical journals and in the popular press mentioned not one word about the vital factor which could and did prevent the aging process!

Yes, as if you didn't already know, it was Vitamin E!

First we should understand something of the methods Selye uses to produce old age. He does it by injecting the rat with a substance, which, if given in immense quantities, is known to cause calcification of the various organs and tissues. There are several substances which can produce "old age" in this fashion; Selye speeded up the process. The heart, the kidneys, and the muscles are among the first to show the effects of old age.

Now, all the rats in this particular experiment which were given the toxic substances (including huge doses of Vitamin D3, parathyroid hormone, and then metallic salts) showed (when autopsied) very obvious "grayish-yellow and somewhat protruding patches" throughout their bodies. Dr. Selye gave the same toxic substance to the other rats, but he had also included a daily dose of Vitamin E, 1,000 mg., a tremendous amount for rats.

When all of the rats were autopsied on the twelfth day, only *one* Vitamin E-treated rat had a small area of "old age patch." All the other *Vitamin E-treated* rats *were normal.* Yet, as we have stated, all of the *non-*Vitamin E-treated rats showed the old age pattern and would have died very shortly, had they not been sacrificed.

In still another phase of the experiment, Selye found that Vitamin E "almost completely inhibited the cardiopathy [heart disease]. It also greatly diminished the nephrocalcinosis (excess calcium in the kidney) and completely inhibited the aortic calcification that accompanied the cardiac lesions." As a clincher to the efficacy of Vitamin E therapy, 90 per cent of the untreated animals died while *every one* of the Vitamin E-treated rats lived.

What more can we say? There is much more evidence, much more proof in Dr. Selye's report, but we do not have the space here to go into any greater detail. If your doctor wishes to read it (as we hope he does), it is listed in the Bibliography.

INDOLENT ULCERS

This condition is more common than is supposed, but it is not common enough to warrant reporting in detail the clear-cut record of approximately fifty reports from many countries where both Vitamin E ointment and oral ingestion were used. The rationale as to why Vitamin E should work in these conditions has already been explained. The interested reader should consult Appendix A, page 152 for bibliographical references.

VARICOSE VEINS

Vitamin E, in massive dosages, according to the Drs. Shute (Appendix A, p. 154) "increases collateral circulation around the deep, obstructed veins, decreases ankle oedema [swelling] and leg ache, halts the varicose process, cuts down or relieves any associated skin irritation, and lets the patient walk much better. Often the veins seem to regress, although this is unpredictable."

The Shutes were among the first to observe the beneficent effect of Vitamin E on varicose veins. This condition is often the forerunner of indolent ulcer. The Shutes' findings are corroborated by other researchers. They do not recommend operations for varicose veins as the same condition usually returns in about one-and-one-half years' time. Why shouldn't it return? The operation admittedly does not clear up the basic cause of varicose veins; it merely removes temporarily the discomfort and unsightly appearances. As the *cause* still exists, the condition, along with the symptoms, usually returns. However, the Shutes agree that, for cosmetic reasons, the operation should be performed if a woman wants it, even though knowing that the condition will probably recur shortly. Now, although the following possibility is not mentioned by the Shutes, why shouldn't a person have the unsightly veins removed by surgery, all the while undertaking a course of Vitamin E therapy? There is every reason to believe that although Vitamin E cannot make new veins out of old, or at least cannot usually remove the unsightliness, it should be able to prevent the return of varicosity by removing at least part of the basic causes. It would be interesting to see this idea carried out by clinical tests.

OTHER DISEASES

There are so many other diseases and disorders which have reportedly been controlled by Vitamin E that we cannot detail all of them here. Knowing the rationale of how Vitamin E functions in every cell, you should have no difficulty in deducing that the vitamin should be of assistance in most of the maladies afflicting mankind. Or animals, for that matter.

We list these diseases or ailments in the next few pages. References for their inclusion are in the Appendix or Bibliography. Also please remember that, in most cases, Vitamin E alone is not to be considered a cure, if indeed there is room in the modern medical lexicon for such a word. The words which should be used in relation to Vitamin E, or any other therapy, are *control* or *partial control, regression* (of the disorder), *benefit, relief* (objective and subjective). Possibly the emphasis on medicine of the future will be prevention rather than cure, for if we knew how to stop a disease before it had a chance to gain a beachhead in the body and/or mind, we would stand a much better chance of living at least to our naturally allotted biological age, generally accepted to be from 120 to 150.

Here are a few of those conditions—heretofore not detailed —and which, statistically speaking, are relatively unimportant but which, as we have mentioned, are a matter of life or death to the victims, their relatives, and friends.

MUSCULAR DYSTROPHY

A good percentage of the victims of muscular dystrophy are benefited by massive dosages of Vitamin E. Some can even achieve retrogression of the disease. But let us emphasize: as yet, Vitamin E, in the present form of administration, has not proved to be a cure or even an efficient controller for most victims of MD. It does benefit *some* sufferers, but a vast amount of research needs to be done. But it is a most promising therapy for muscular dystrophy which should be explored systematically. (See Bibliography: Beckman; Castelar; Pinheiro; De Carlo, *et al.;* Gimlette; Rovetta and Bonaretti; Nielsen and Marvin; Gros and Kirnberger; Shcherbakova.)

ARTHRITIS

There are many types of arthritis—rheumatoid, polyarthritis, osteoarthritis, to mention the three most common forms. Vitamin E in massive dosages has proven of benefit in several forms of arthritis. Patients feel better, mobility of the joints is improved, and pain is reduced or eliminated in some cases. Vitamin E alone, however, is not claimed to be more than an aid to arthritics. The reports are numerous; they cannot be enumerated here, but among them are Barwick-Schramm and Dumanska.

MONGOLIAN IDIOCY

Now here is a disease of youngsters which creates a sympathetic response in everyone because it is so tragic for the parents. Not tragic for the youngster, of course, as he is completely unaware of what is going on. Medicine says there is no cure and no hope for these unfortunate children who are born with an affliction of the brain which dooms them to idiocy as long as they live. (Some may live for quite a while without ever being aware of their environment.) Until Dr. A. Del Giudice, Chief of Child Psychology, National Institute of Public Health, Buenos Aires, Argentina, and Dr. Anna Szasz of Budapest, Hungary, began their important experiments with Vitamin E combined with Vitamin C, there was no hope for these illfated children. Yet by administering daily 2,000 to 3,000 units (2 to 3 grams) of Vitamin E together with an equivalent amount of Vitamin C, the researchers were able to obtain remarkable effects in the disease which is "known" to be incurable. (If you have a child with Mongolian idiocy, then you should look up the appropriate references, obtain a copy of them, and confront your doctor with the proof. That is probably your only hope. Your doctor, of course, will tell you there is no hope and probably would not look up the references himself since he has been told that Vitamin E doesn't work on *any* of man's ailments. And how could it possibly work on such an obscure, hopeless affliction as Mongolian idiocy?)

KIDNEY DISEASES

Many researchers, including the Drs. Shute, have found that Vitamin E, in sufficient dosages, clears up or controls many forms of kidney disease, including *nephritis,* one of the most common forms. The literature on this subject is voluminous. The general consensus of most of the researchers is that Vitamin E produces *diuresis* (improved kidney function) thereby reducing excess water in the tissues. Further, the vitamin exerts a beneficent effect on the kidney cells themselves. We do not have space to present details here, but the interested reader may refer to the Bibliography.[29]

LIVER DISEASE

There is much evidence, both animal and human, that Vitamin E aids in restoring the functions of damaged livers. Among the researchers responsible for these findings on humans is Dr. V. Bonomini of the University of Bologna, Italy. He reported treating thirty-one patients with various liver ailments and obtained good to excellent results except in two cases with far-advanced cirrhosis complicated by *ascites* (abdominal swelling). All four cases of chronic pre-cirrhotic liver disease were greatly benefited, both objectively and subjectively. Especially interesting were Dr. Bonomini's findings on eleven patients with

[29] Shute, E. V.; Shute, W. E.; Prosperi; Klotz and Debray; O'Connor; Medina; Comi; Butturini; Becker-Freysang; Dinda; Bellotti *et al.;* Accornero; Kunstmann; Emmel; Choudbury and Nandi; Delinotte and Vonthron; Mervyn and Morton; Suardi.

diabetes whose livers were swollen and mal-functioning. All showed excellent results, proved by many tests, including the fact that their insulin requirement was reduced 40–60 per cent within 25 to 30 days! (This corroborates other researchers' findings on Vitamin E's therapeutic efficacy in treating diabetes, which we have mentioned previously.) Dr. Bonomini classifies Vitamin E as a "hepatoprotective" (liver-protective) drug. His observations are also corroborated by Dr. F. Wennig, of Graz, Austria, among others. (See Beckman; Stormont, *et al.;* Hadnagy, *et al.;* Rodnan, *et al.*)

PEPTIC ULCER

Dr. J. Canto Soler, of Spain, writing in a Spanish journal of nutrition (see Bibliography), reported on the treatment of 188 peptic ulcer sufferers. He injected them daily (until pain was relieved) with 100 milligrams of alpha tocopherol. He obtained excellent results in 115 patients, good results in 25; apparently there was no effect in the remaining 30 (except the lessening or disappearance of pain). Dr. M. K. Horwitt (previously noted) of the Elgin State Hospital, Elgin, Ill., and the University of Illinois College of Medicine in Chicago, in a monumental five-year controlled study of Vitamin E requirements in humans, was surprised when a Vitamin-E deficient diet *produced* peptic ulcers in his volunteers. This finding would seem to confirm that lack of Vitamin E does have an adverse effect on the gastro-intestinal tract to the point of causing ulcers, and the ulcers may be treated successfully with the proper doses of Vitamin E.

We need go no further into the other multifarious benefits of Vitamin E. The reader by this time certainly should be able to ascertain its universal action in almost every disease known to man and/or animals. These include disorders of the gastro-intestinal tract (Fajer, *et al.*), also such diseases as chronic poliomyelitis (Jacques; E. V. Shute), leprosy (De Campos Magalhaes and Figueiredo Barbosa; Sarmento; Bergel; Floch and Horth; Mason and Bergel), diseases of the eye (Desusclade;

Sbordone; Vannas and Orma) and skin (Walther; Nikolowski; Frey; Grubb; Kimmig)—even psoriasis. Researchers usually treat these conditions with other vitamins and supplements in conjunction with Vitamin E. As we have repeatedly pointed out, Vitamin E should be used in conjunction with other vitamins and food supplements to obtain best results. And, as we have also repeatedly reported, almost all the orthodox, "authoritative," medical agencies will tell you or your doctor that Vitamin E is of little or no value in either the prevention or control of any of the ailments we have mentioned.

7

Communications and Vitamin E

This writer is only one among many thousands who have been saved by the indomitable Drs. Shute and their teams of researchers at the Shute Foundation. Another one among those thousands was J. I. Rodale, manufacturer of electrical devices and now the founder-editor of *Prevention* magazine. *Prevention*, under editor Rodale's guidance, has grown from nothing but a dream thirteen years ago to become one of America's leading health magazines, with a guaranteed paid circulation of about 350,000. Of course, the magazine reaches many more readers than the actual circulation figure: it is passed to many friends and relatives. It is one of the very few popular publications in this country which is in the vanguard of new, valid medical research. *Prevention* has several eminent researchers on its staff, including W. J. McCormick, M.D. In over 90 per cent of its articles, the magazine cites for its authority medical researchers from all over the world.

Editor Rodale has furnished us with an excellent description of how he was saved by the Shutes and Vitamin E. His was an early case of angina—but the story is best told in his own words from the June, 1961, issue of *Prevention:*

Vitamin E is one of the strongest planks in our [*Prevention*] program because in this lethargic age there is an alarming reduction in the body's supply of oxygen, and vitamin E has the effect of oxygenation of the tissues. This is a matter of life and death when it comes to the action of the heart.

I first heard of the Shutes' work with vitamin E in 1940 when

Time magazine was so good as to announce their work and their claims. At that time I was experiencing slight angina chest pains on exertion. I had a heart condition since boyhood, but the doctors evidently didn't want to scare me by telling me. In 1921 Life Extension Institute told me I had a heart murmur, but in the early 1950's I was turned down for life insurance on account of a bad electrocardiogram.

But in 1940 I am sure that the Shutes saved my life, and I herewith wish to acknowledge my gratefulness to them and to their brave attitude and strong resistance to the whole medical profession, which evidently must have seen economic danger were this vitamin to be widely adopted. They fought the Shutes tooth and nail, with no holds barred, depending on their usual statement, "There is no evidence" when there were mountains of evidence.

At any rate, I bought my first bottle of vitamin E capsules in 1940, which was made by Squibb, and noted that it was derived from vegetable oils. At that time I was not aware of any distinction between a natural or a synthetic source, but I began by taking 100 milligrams per day (mixed tocopherols) as the bottle stated. And they had a miraculous effect. My angina pains went down quite a bit. The label said to take 100 milligrams daily, or as directed by a physician. I then began to take 200 milligrams a day, and I began to feel a little better. Slowly I raised my daily intake until about 5 years ago it reached 1,200 milligrams a day, and this gave me what I needed to control my angina fully.

Once I went up to the Shutes' clinic in Canada for a full checkup, and Dr. Evan Shute checked upon my daily dosage. However, the Shutes favor the alpha tocopherol form of vitamin E, rather than the mixed tocopherols. I, therefore, began to take the alpha tocopherol and some of my angina pains returned. This may be a personal idiosyncrasy. People should find out for themselves by trial which form is best.

The mixed tocopherols consist of 4 types of tocopherols i.e., alpha, beta, delta, and gamma. I get my alpha from the mixed batch. The alpha is about 60% of the total. The less fragmentation I get, the better I like it. Nature mixed the tocopherols together, perhaps for a purpose. At any rate, Dr. Shute told me that for the best effect, the body must be saturated with the vitamin. The only indication against taking large doses of vitamin E is where one has high blood pressure. Then perhaps one shouldn't take more than 300 of the mixed tocopherols [except under medical care].

I have been taking vitamin E now for about 21 years, and I am sure it is keeping me from having a heart attack. Our family has a history of heart disease. My father died of it at age 51, my oldest brother at 51, my next oldest at 62, Joe at 56, Tina at 64, and Sally at 60. In August I will be 63 years old and can walk miles with ease, thanks to my vitamin E, and of course also to my whole Prevention program. But without vitamin E I couldn't do it. There is no reason why I can't reach 100 unless I am killed in an accident. I would love to have the last laugh over the insurance company that I will have beat out of so many unearned premiums. [Editor Rodale is now 65 and going stronger than ever.]

There is one effect of vitamin E that I would like to talk about. It is a non-health effect. I believe it has greatly increased my mental efficiency. There are many persons who are not health-conscious. Under no condition would they ever take a vitamin to make them feel better or live longer. They want none of it. They want to be normal. But if they realized that by taking this vitamin they would be able to get more out of their brain then perhaps they would take it.

I reiterate that this vitamin should increase mental efficiency, because the textbooks state that vitamin E is an oxygen conserver—it oxygenates all the miles of veins, arteries, nerves, etc., that go into every part of the body—even into the brain. I can see it in the terrific increase in my mental capacity, which has improved at least 300% since I began taking vitamin E in 1940. It shows in the amount of mental work I can do today at age 63. And the future of my mental front looks very bright indeed. I believe that this vitamin will be a potent factor in keeping off doddering senility, which is due more or less to the slowing down of the circulation, the smaller delivery of oxygen to the various avenues and arteries of the body.

From our correspondence we know that thousands have helped themselves to a better heart condition and to other improvements in health by taking vitamin E.

The following is a random sampling of the correspondence.

VITAMIN E FOR THROMBOPHLEBITIS

A wonderful letter from Forrest J. Caldwell of Illinois tells us of his experience using vitamin E for thrombophlebitis. "I want to thank and praise you for the article on phlebitis and vitamin E. I have been taking vitamin E now for 30 days. My case started with an attack in 1936. My legs were 22 inches around, my entire body increased to half again its normal size up to my ribs. I have had 16 doctors including the Mayo Clinic. My doctor always said if someone could give me a new set of legs I'd be okay. He wanted to tie off the veins. At the Mayo Clinic they wanted to cut in above and below the knee and tie off the veins. I would not permit it.

"After treatment with vitamin E the blood clots are gone, my legs are normal. I have no swelling or gangerene signs. I cannot say enough. There are no words to express my gratitude. This is a Godsend. I am 62 years of age and I never felt better in my life, after 30 days of religious treatment with vitamin E."

SWOLLEN ANKLES IMPROVE

Here is a letter from W. V. A. Franklin of Los Angeles, California, who says: "It was last October that I heard of vitamin E, in *Prevention,* I think. At that time I had swollen ankles and aching legs and knees. I began to take vitamin E. The swollen ankles and aching leg pains disappeared. My shortness of breath, so bad I was obliged to keep my sleeping room wide open, disappeared. Now I can sleep with the house closed up if I want to. My heart beats more constantly than before, when it used to miss every other beat at times."

VITAMIN E FOR HYPERTENSION

Another subscriber from San Antonio, Texas, who prefers to remain anonymous, says, "Vitamin E as prescribed by Dr. Shute has reduced my hypertension to normal limits thereby cheating the surgeon out of another statistic!

"I am currently taking 450 milligrams daily and as a result am no longer annoyed with angina pectoris, shortage of breath, extremely high blood pressure and other cardiac disturbances. I have used vitamin E under Dr. Shute's prescribed dosage for the past 15 months. I go up and down stairs easily, walk any distance I desire up hill and down and can perform the run-of-mill chores around the home without any cardiac embarrassment. This was not possible prior to the vitamin E therapy.

"I have had high blood pressure for years as well as angina, and prior to vitamin E treatment experienced 3 attacks of coronary thrombosis. Vitamin E is the best insurance policy I have found and with due regard for my limitations and all attending factors such as proper diet, rest and so forth, I hope to live out my allotted span in wholesome comfort."

VITAMIN CURES VARICOSE VEINS

Walter Weck, Jr., of Long Branch, New Jersey, recently sent us some information on the wonders of vitamin E. Says he: "One of my wife's friends developed very bad varicose veins early in her second pregnancy and after delivery one leg swelled up with phlebitis. Eventually she submitted to having her veins injected by her doctor and had the usual immediate relief. However, almost immediately after becoming pregnant the third time, the swollen veins reappeared, worse than before! Leg cramps would develop every day late in the afternoon, and she had to be off her feet completely in the evening. We suggested 'E.' Her doctor neither approved or disapproved, so she tried it. Within 3 days the aching had eased and by the end of the first week of vitamin E, the swollen veins had all but disappeared."

A SYSTOLIC CONDITION RELIEVED

From Mrs. F. Louis Koenig of Milwaukee, Wisconsin, comes the following communication: "After our local doctors—heart specialists specifically, plus two doctors in the heart clinic at Rochester, Minnesota—had advised me that I would just have to learn to live with a systolic heart condition, I found out about the Shute Institute through an article of yours. I wrote them for information in July, 1953. I began to take vitamin E immediately, and as of January first or thereabouts I no longer have any systoles—in fact, I seem absolutely cured and never felt better in my life. It has been perhaps one of the most amazing experiences of my life, to say nothing of the relief and satisfaction."

VITAMIN E BENEFITS EVERYONE

Another letter on vitamin E and the almost miraculous results obtained from taking it: "Dear Mr. Rodale: My wife suffered for over a year with severe heart palpitations which would awaken her from a sound sleep at night. The doctor said there was nothing wrong with the heart but still the symptoms continued. Then she tried vitamin E and within a week the palpitations were gone and have stayed gone. She is continuing with the vitamin E nevertheless, because of the benefits to the vascular system. This same vitamin played a strange trick on us; an external examination a year ago indicated a fibrosed and hardening uterus—probably no more children. Our third child is expected to arrive this summer, very probably thanks to vitamin E.

"My brother-in-law had a slight heart attack which showed some damage to the heart. Since then he has had dizzy spells whenever hard pressed at work, could not stay awake in the evenings and generally was not himself. We suggested vitamin E. Today the dizzy spells are non-existent, his vitality has returned, and his wife complains she can't get him to go to bed!

"My mother-in-law had her leg up on a chair most of the summer as a result of phlebitis; the doctor said that was all she could do—just sit and wait. We suggested vitamin E. A week later the swelling was gone. When she ran out of the vitamin E, she gave it a try without, just to see what would happen. Within a few days the leg began to swell again, only to subside once more when she returned to vitamin E."

VITAMIN E AND HEART DISEASE

Mrs. George Wilson of 1711½ John Avenue, Superior, Wisconsin, writes us about the benefits she received from taking vitamin E. Says she: "I must mention that through *Prevention* I read of the Drs. Shute in Canada and their work with vitamin E for the heart. As I have an injured heart, I took a trip there last June to have them prescribe for me. They did and I am so glad and happy to say they helped me wonderfully. How AMA can hold back on recommending it is more than I can understand."

Editor Rodale's beneficial experience with Vitamin E proved to be the means of saving many other thousands of persons. In June, 1950, he began publication of *Prevention,* and therewith, among other things, Rodale's personal Vitamin E crusade was launched. Fortunately, he had the money, the stamina, and, most important, the courage. He brought to his ever-increasing readership the also constantly increasing accumulation of favorable reports throughout the world of the magic vitamin. And, as we have mentioned, Rodale, even as does the present writer, owes his life to Vitamin E.

Meanwhile, in another medium, an eminent nutritionist, Carlton Fredericks, Ph.D., has also been enlightening radio audiences, which number in the millions, about the values of Vitamin E. Dr. Fredericks is in the forefront of every battle to bring the truth about health, nutrition, and medical research to his listeners. At this writing, Dr. Fredericks is carried five days a week over more than 200 radio stations. His audience is fanatically devoted, especially since many of them, including this writer, have derived untold benefits from his vast facilities for coordinating research from all over the world and making the research available. Otherwise, extremely important findings would be buried, as they usually are, until someone of the calibre of Fredericks digs them out and makes the authorities eat humble pie.

Now there are others who would also expose the Tiger at our Gates. There is the magazine called *Herald of Health,* which, while not nearly so large and influential as Rodale's *Prevention,* nevertheless does its share of informing the public on the truth about Vitamin E, among other things. While you may not subscribe whole-heartedly to everything *Herald of Health* reports, remember that the Tiger is defeated only by a concerted, joint effort. The magazine *Truth* is also bringing the true story of Vitamin E to its readers.

Another publication which has been doing a remarkable job in Washington and elsewhere is the *National Health Federation Bulletin.* This is the monthly periodical issued by the National Health Federation, which group, to my mind, is the leading organization—with a lobby in Washington—attempting to maintain freedom in the healing arts. I would advise anyone interested in preserving our traditional freedoms in matters of health and medicine to join the National Health Federation.

8

What You Can Do to Help Yourself and Others

If you suffer from cardiovascular disease or from any disease mentioned in this book which Vitamin E has proved to be of value in controlling, then you are probably under the care of a physician. And you are probably *not* receiving Vitamin E.

Our first suggestion would be to show your doctor this book. Ask him to read it regardless of preconceived notions concerning Vitamin E therapy. After reading the book, the doctor should write for the latest literature available from the Shute Foundation, 10 Grand Avenue, London, Ontario, Canada. Also he should obtain the latest copies of the Annotated Bibliography of Vitamin E which has been compiled periodically by the National Vitamin Foundation, 250 West 57th Street, New York, N.Y., since 1940; they are invaluable for a doctor wishing to learn the truth about Vitamin E.

These compilations on Vitamin E are truly scientific in that they encompass every phase of Vitamin E's activity so that no doctor and/or scientist should be confused by the material presented. For instance, here are some of the division headings on Vitamin E:

> Occurrence and Distribution
> Determination (Physical, Chemical)
> Chemistry
> Physiology and Pathology (including the Circulatory
>   System: heart, vascular system, and blood)

> Pharmacology
> Nutrition and Metabolism
> Medical and Therapeutic Use

Their last category includes:

> Diseases of Infants and Prematures
> Disorders of the Muscles, Bones, Joints, Connective Tissue, and Collagen
> Nervous System and Neuromuscular Disorders
> Diseases of Liver, Kidney, and Gastrointestinal Tract
> Cardiovascular Diseases and Blood Dyscrasias [abnormalities in the blood]
> Allergies and Diseases of the Skin
> Obstetrics and Gynecology [Various abnormal conditions are presented here that have been treated successfully with Vitamin E therapy. They include: spontaneous abortion, toxaemias of pregnancy, menopausal and menstrual disorders, sterility and fertility.]
> Ophthalmology; Otology, Dental, and Oral Disorders
> Endocrine Dysfunctions
> Malnutrition, Infections, and Metabolic Effects

After reading this present work, its appendices and bibliography, and after reviewing the material from the Vitamin Foundation, your doctor should have no doubts about Vitamin E's value. Should all this fail to convince him, our next recommendation is that you visit the Shute Clinic in London, Ontario, Canada. I have learned that their charges are minimal and that very likely the money you are spending now would be no more than the cost of a trip to Canada. Further, you would have the expert supervision of those doctors who know most about the dosage and general care of Vitamin E-treated patients. After careful investigation I can almost guarantee that the fees charged would be less or comparable to the fees that you are now paying in the United States.[30]

---

[30] While we are on the subject of fees, let us scotch a particularly vicious rumor about Dr. E. V. Shute. The rumor, as told to me and

However, if you cannot visit the Shute Clinic and if your own doctor refuses to supervise your treatment with Vitamin E, what are you to do? Our advice is to find another doctor, one who is enlightened enough to recognize the *harmlessness* of the treatment even if he has no confidence in its efficacy. Refer him to the authoritative and universally accepted *Taber's Cyclopedic Medical Dictionary* (1963 Edition, Ninth Edition) which not only pronounces alpha tocopherol "non-toxic even in large doses," but under *Uses,* states without equivocation: "In heart cases including coronary thrombosis; a preventive of heart conditions; in Buerger's disease; in hemorrhage." And further, under *Action,* it states: "Decreases oxygen requirements of heart muscles 50 per cent or more, increasing blood supply. Decreases excessive capillary permeability, or leakage; reduces blood clot in a thrombus, or prevents its formation and softens scar tissue."

Now what more authority could your doctor ask for? But

widely circulated in medical groups, is that Dr. Shute is "making a fortune from the sale of Vitamin E capsules"; that he has "a considerable share of stock in a pharmaceutical house which manufactures Vitamin E." An investigation proved these rumors to be absolutely without foundation, as I had suspected from previous investigation of rumors concerning famous (and controversial) medical men. If their methods and their evidence are unassailable, then the orthodox attack the man personally. The "authorities" spread rumors that he is either a homosexual, a Communist, or a former Nazi, that he is a narcotic addict or, particularly in medicine, that he obtained his M.D. under questionable circumstances, or that he now is suffering from cerebral arteriosclerosis and, therefore, is not capable of making scientific judgments. Or, worse, that the whole method he advocates is just a big "money-making" scheme. The latter approach is the most ironic of all since most of the officials who indulge in such chicanery are themselves the recipients of salaries, grants, and other emoluments which far exceed the income of the accused.

After many years of dedicated work, Dr. E. V. Shute was granted by the non-profit Shute Foundation an annual salary of approximately $23,000, no stock holdings, no deals of any kind. This is a figure which most specialists would sneer at, particularly those who have spent their lifetime at their specialty and have gained a world-wide reputation. Such a rumor is unfortunate because I believe a man of Dr. Shute's calibre should be rewarded for his work, not subjected to such dishonest accusations.

if he still is sceptical or concerned, there is a third procedure I can recommend: that is for you to purchase Vitamin E (it can be bought at any drug store, health food store, or vitamin mail order house without a prescription since it is classified by the FDA as a non-toxic vitamin, not a drug) and start taking Vitamin E on your own.

Except in extremely rare instances, Vitamin E (alpha tocopherol), in normal dosages, is absolutely without adverse side effects. In a few patients—usually those with a history of a rare type of high blood pressure—*large initial* doses of Vitamin E may tend to raise the pressure temporarily. Then it drops again; in fact, Vitamin E, when taken over a period of time actually acts as a hypotensive (a blood pressure lowering agent) in some patients. (See Appendix A, p. 141 and Appendix C.)

However, in view of the fact that even one person in a million may experience temporary side-effects from ingesting large dosages of Vitamin E, most researchers advise beginning with a dose which cannot possibly produce side-reactions of any sort. This dosage is generally acknowledged by most recent investigators to be about 100 international units per day (100 mg.). After the first two weeks, the dosage is gradually increased week by week until the optimum relief is obtained. Such a small initial dosage may not achieve the desired results for some persons for some time (occasionally six months to a year!), but since we are not giving medical advice, in the interests of those very rare persons who may respond initially to the larger dosages with temporarily raised blood pressure, it is better to begin with the smaller dosage and then gradually raise it to the optimum. The optimum may be as high as 800 to 1,000 units. Let us now state emphatically that no fatalities or even ill effects have been reported from even large doses of the vitamin. (If so, it would be in the voluminous literature and be noted by the AMA, FDA, *et al.*)

Of course, if you could obtain a physician who would supervise your therapy, then he would probably start you off on 150 or 200 I.U. units and build up from there. In my own case, I began on my own with 600 units daily and am now taking 1,500 I.U. and sometimes even more.

Remember, we have been speaking of persons who are already under a doctor's care for cardiovascular illnesses. Researchers in Vitamin E believe that the so-called "normal" person can ward off a potential manifestation of cardiovascular disease by taking 100 I.U. per day as a start and then building up to an average of 400 to 600 units for the average-size woman and 600 to 800 for the average-size man. The Drs. Shute are among those researchers who are quite sure (on the basis of the curative results as well as the provable increase in heart function in "normals") that the larger dosages are the most effective. The Shutes have written that if they have erred in Vitamin E therapy in the past, it was in giving too small a dose in the beginning. Now, Dr. Shute writes he would have put many of his early patients on a much higher dosage had he known then what he knows now.

The reader may have observed that many researchers are combining Vitamin E therapy with Vitamin A and, frequently, calcium. Others are using Vitamin C and inositol (one of the Vitamin B-complex group) as well as other factors. There is much evidence to demonstrate that vitamins should always be used in combination since vitamins work in conjunction with one another, with hormones, and with enzyme systems. Further, many vitamins are actually *antagonists* of each other; over-simplified, this means that if the body obtains more than it can utilize of a particular vitamin, certain other vitamins or substances (if present) will counteract the overabundance effect of the first vitamin. Usually, however, a superabundance of a vitamin is eliminated without harm to the body. The exceptions are Vitamins A and D, which have been shown to be toxic when given in huge quantities for a long period of time. However, recent studies have demonstrated that if these vitamins had not been given alone (which they were) but had been accompanied by other vitamins and *minerals,* with which most vitamins have to combine in order to be effective (and to destroy superfluous amounts of any vitamin), their toxicity would have been non-existent or at least greatly reduced. As reported many times and acknowledged by all authorities, Vitamin E, along with Vitamin C and many others, has been demonstrated to be non-toxic per se, even when unaccompanied by treatment with other vitamins.

However, in lieu of medical supervision, you would be prudent to include a multi-vitamin and mineral capsule along with the Vitamin E. Also, since it has been found by some researchers that calcium may enhance E's effect, and you cannot actually obtain enough calcium except by drinking a quart of milk daily or by eating a quarter-pound of the regular cheeses, researchers suggest either calcium tablets of bone meal, dicalcium phosphate, or crushed oyster shell tablets.

And because Vitamin C is so essential to the permeability and "integrity" of the capillary walls—working in some fashion with Vitamin E in that respect—many doctors acquainted with nutrition (for example, Dr. Hirsch) recommend an extra supplement of Vitamin C in addition to their concomitants, the bioflavonoids—substances found commonly in the pulp and connective tissues of fruits. Friends of mine and I take at least 3,000 units of Vitamin C and bioflavonoids daily. We also take supplements of the B-complex because we believe, contrary to the FDA reports, the human need for vitamins is actually much greater than recommended by these agencies—since there really is no "normal average" American diet. The combined effect has been impressive.

Everyone nowadays is familiar with the American Medical Association's attempt to deride all vitamin-taking as a mere waste of time and money. The propaganda asserts that the normal American, eating a normal diet, obtains enough vitamins and minerals and that any more that are ingested are eliminated without benefit to the recipient. This campaign against vitamins and other supplements by the AMA and, consequently, its stooges in the U.S. Government such as the FDA, is rendered even more ridiculous when, conversely, the pages of the *Journal of the American Medical Association* are filled with advertising for vitamins. The ads cite study after study in which vitamins have been used with great benefit and in which doctors are urged to prescribe them to their patients. And, of course, the *JAMA* is filled with research articles about the necessity of extra vitamins under almost every condition one could imagine. Naturally, as we may begin to suspect, the extra vitamins are not effective *except when prescribed by a physician,* who also, naturally, prescribes the specific vitamins as advertised in the pages of AMA journal.

In other words, extra vitamins are worthless except when specifically prescribed by an M.D.—who will usually not prescribe them—and compounded by an "ethical" pharmaceutical house which advertises in the AMA's official publications. These vitamins so compounded cost you about three times as much as when purchased through a vitamin mail-order house. Yet, as almost anyone knows who has made a study of the problem, 80 per cent of all the vitamins manufactured in the United States are manufactured by the gigantic U.S. Vitamin Corporation.

This corporation supplies the various pharmaceutical houses with the basic vitamin products; the pharmaceutical houses, in turn, attach their own labels and, in many instances, *put a different coating on the pill* in order to differentiate *their* product from the others. The exact formulation (such as how much B, or C, or A comprises their particular brand) is the prerogative of the company buying the vitamin product, and they will make every endeavor to disguise the fact that the original vitamin material was bought elsewhere.

Therefore, without delving further into the ethics of the AMA, which is definitely fighting for their "in" group much more than a labor union ever fought automation, let us continue with how you and I can save ourselves from heart disease in spite of the organized propaganda to the contrary.

As we stated before, the important factor in *recognized*

heart disease is building up to the optimum dosages of Vitamin E, along with other vitamins and minerals. The optimum dosage of Vitamin E is that which is effective for *you*. Remember that each person is different; some demand high doses of about anything while others need little of exactly the same material. This is due to heredity, stress (sometimes classified as environment), and differing absorption ratios. With regard to the latter factor, some persons may absorb only 10 per cent of any vitamin they take; others may absorb 20 to 30 per cent. Absorption of any food or vitamin depends, for the most part, on the state of the individual, usually the condition of the intestines, where the entrance of nutrients into the bloodstream is effected.

As for Vitamin E's non-toxicity—even in what must be considered tremendous dosages—Dr. Del Giudice of Argentina has given mentally retarded children 2,000 to 3,000 units of Vitamin E daily for many years with excellent results and with no evidence of toxicity. (We have already examined Dr. Del Giudice's studies in Chapter 6 under Mongolian Idiocy.) One volunteer in the U.S. took two to four grams (2,000 to 4,000 mg. or I.U.) every day for three months without any noticeable adverse side reactions. Four grams is 4,000 units of Vitamin E—about four times the dosage prescribed for the "average" heart patient.

To sum up the situation as to what you should do whether you are a heart and/or cardiovascular disease patient or whether you wish to prevent being such a patient, the best scientific advice to date is:

1. Take supplementary capsules of Vitamin E, starting with 100 units and building up the intake gradually until you can detect a definite improvement in your well-being. Also, take a multi-vitamin-mineral capsule, B-complex, calcium, and Vitamin C in conjunction with bioflavonoids.

2. Begin a regular program of exercise. Do not, of course, exercise too heavily at first, but allow at least one hour (or if possible) two hours a day for a planned regime. This could

take the form of bicycle riding as advocated by Dr. Paul Dudley White, but if you don't have a bicycle or the facilities for riding one, do gymnastic exercises in your home. Or you could walk very rapidly around the block, building up to six or eight times. Most sports and games are excellent; swimming is one of the best forms of exercise in that almost all the muscles of the body are used, yet none to great excess. The Canadian Air Force system of exercise has been reported to be excellent, particularly for those who can spend only a limited amount of exercise time a day. Also, Dr. John A. Faulkner of the University of Michigan has developed a remarkable system of exercise but which, in the main, needs to be conducted under professional supervision. (See Bibliography.)

3. It would probably be wise in lieu of our lack of knowledge as to what causes heart attacks not to eat too many fats (or too much of other foods) unless you are able to metabolize them by violent or semi-violent exercise. The eating of fats has probably acquired a disproportionate role in medical and public thinking during the past ten to fifteen years. However, since the reports on cholesterol, fats, etc., are now consistently contradictory as we have seen, it might be wise to withhold judgment. A year or so ago, it was very fashionable in most medical circles to blame cholesterol and animal fats as *the* cause of heart disease. Now, it is not so wise to attach the blame solely to cholesterol since it has been found to be a most essential substance in human metabolism; indeed the body manufactures its own. Further, as we have pointed out previously, cholesterol is not the initial villain in instituting the first atherosclerotic plaques laid down on the *intima*—the lining of the blood vessels. Another form of fats—tryglycerides—has been indicted now as the real culprit in the initial arteriosclerotic process by a number of researchers (or so they say now). Yet no one knows the way this actually happens. As we have indicated previously, if fats, carbohydrates, or any one dietary factor were really the sole cause of heart disease in all peoples under all circumstances, then the other parts of the

world would be in the same unenviable position in relation to heart disease as the U.S.

Although the American Medical Association has not yet recognized Vitamin E as an agent for treating cardiovascular diseases, it, officially, has not swung along with the popular tide of anti-cholesterol, anti-fat diets which have been sweeping the country for the last ten years. The *Journal of the AMA* has printed articles both *pro* and *con* on the subject, and editorially the AMA journal has not taken an absolute stand. It is to its credit that the editorial board of the JAMA recognizes—in spite of its shortcomings on other issues—that a true controversy exists among medical men concerning the role of cholesterol and the ingestion of other fats. They have taken a moderate, even scientific attitude until the issue is settled by proper experiments and studies. They will find that this attitude should have been adopted in every field of their endeavors; then they would not be fighting in the popular and scientific plane to maintain their "image" among the people; and they would not have to spend millions of dollars to maintain this image both in public communications and in lobbying in Washington.

Let us point out that if you are undertaking the "unsaturated" fat diet which has been promulgated by several popular books on dieting in recent years, you ought to be informed that unsaturated fats take quite a bit of Vitamin E out of the body. In fact, Horwitt, *et al.*, Harris, *et al.*, among others, state that the need for Vitamin E is often increased *six-fold* if a person consumes large amounts of unsaturated fats (see Bibliography).

The body (and what we call the mind) lives in a constant state of chemical change. Vitamins, minerals, enzymes, and other substances in the blood both accentuate and negate each other's actions so that each cell is kept in a state of dynamic equilibrium, constantly changing each ten trillionth of a second to suit its own needs and that of the body as a whole. This "desire" and the workings of the body for such optimal "normal" equilibrium is termed "homeostasis." The efforts of the

body to maintain the normal represent a picture of such continual, instantaneous reactions that it staggers the brain to think
of the complex processes involved when a trillionth of a second
means the difference between the life or death of a cell.

Nevertheless, in practical terms we now know that Vitamin
E, if taken in sufficient amounts, can help maintain the body's
homeostasis in each cell and that this beneficial action is most
dramatically demonstrated in the heart and blood vessels.

Let us add one more note of advice for athletes. We have
reported previously that Vitamin E enhances the ability of
animals to withstand stresses of all types, to ward off old age,
and to increase their racing and physical prowess. The last
is especially true for athletes.

One of the most conclusive studies originates from West
Germany. Dr. L. Prokop (see Bibliography) conducted a study
of the effect of Vitamin E on oxygen consumption on thirty
men, some of whom were trained athletes. The men ranged in
age from 18 to 54 and were tested during and after violent
exercise. A "control" was established, which as we have seen,
requires the use of a "placebo" so that the men would not
know what they were receiving. The tocopherol or placebo
was administered one hour before exercise for five consecutive
days (the dosage was small: 1 milligram per kilogram of body
weight; for instance, a man weighing 150 pounds received
about 68 milligrams of Vitamin E; however, since the dosage
was by injection, there was naturally more absorption).

Dr. Prokop found that the Vitamin E did not decrease
the need for oxygen during the exercise itself but did decrease
the need for it after the exercise. This is called oxygen "debt":
the tocopherol users did not have to repay to the body in terms
of muscular fatigue what the non-users had to repay. As the
experimenter noted, the lower the oxygen debt incurred, the
better the recovery.

However, since the exercise prescribed by the experimenter
lasted only five minutes, it is more than probable that, had the
test lasted longer, not only would the oxygen debt have been

altered favorably by Vitamin E, but the actual consumption of oxygen during exercise would have also been favorably influenced. Other tests have shown this to be true, particularly in the practical sense. Almost every professional or amateur athlete competing today, who has won honors or set records, uses Vitamin E as well as the other vitamin supplements. Apparently they have not read, or do not trust, the edicts issued by Official Medicine that vitamins and other supplements other than the minimum recommended by the AMA and FDA are of no value and cannot possibly benefit the body in any way.

In "Sporting Comments" a column by E. Mehl, Sports Editor of the *Kansas City Star,* Mehl cites the use of Vitamin E by many famous athletes: Joie Ray, who, on his sixty-fourth birthday, ran a mile in five minutes, 30 seconds and believes he can cut it to five minutes even. He is certain his stamina comes from his use of Vitamin E. Herb Elliott used wheat germ when he was establishing mile records. Eddie Beck who broke the 100-yard junior backstroke record in the National A.A.U. in 1958 is another champion who uses wheat germ, as is Dave Mills of Ohio State who won the 100-yard dash in 9.7 seconds, the 220 in 21.2 seconds, and the 440 in 46.6 seconds.

Eighty-eight per cent of American Olympic Stars use wheat germ; 86 per cent use wheat germ oil (an even richer source of Vitamin E), and 84 per cent use vitamin preparations. Quite a few use all three.

But perhaps the most recent example of an athletic star using Vitamin E is that of Murray Rose, who is the youngest Olympic triple gold medal winner in history. Murray has now won a total of six Olympic medals in distance swimming. Murray's father, in his recent book, *Faith, Love and Seaweed,* reveals the secret of his son's stamina. In addition to rigorous training and plenty of natural talent, Murray eats a special diet which includes every vitamin and mineral known (and no doubt some that have not been identified yet). In addition to wheat germ, brewers' yeast, and rose hips, young Rose takes Vitamin E, particularly on occasions when there is the need for extra muscular exertion, such as a swimming contest. Murray takes from 200 to 1,500 units of Vitamin E. According to the elder Rose, wheat germ and wheat germ oil are rapidly becoming as much a necessity for the daily routine of an athlete as his daily workout.

There are at least three controlled experiments being conducted on human athletes, and perhaps we shall soon see the results. Already preliminary results in Australia, Canada, and Northern Ireland indicate success with Vitamin E. However, it was Dr. A. Goria of Italy (see Bibliography) who performed the classic experiments on normal human subjects using the electrocardiograph (ECG). These experiments prove that Vitamin E can and does improve the function of the "normal" heart as well as aid the circulatory and metabolic systems of the body. Dr. Goria used "before and after" tests; that is, his subjects took Vitamin E for twenty days and were tested with the ECG and then taken off Vitamin E and tested after two months.

Dr. Goria studied many phases of the heart action with the ECG. The primary method he employed was deprivation of oxygen (hypoxia). He had his volunteers breathe a small percentage of oxygen (7.5 per cent) mixed with a large amount of nitrogen (approximately 92.5 per cent) for three minutes. Now, while we know nitrogen is most valuable for growing plants, it does nothing for animals; in fact, heavy concentrations of this "inert" substance without sufficient oxygen will produce death quickly.

When not on Vitamin E, his volunteers experienced "much distress" after about two minutes of breathing this oxygen-poor mixture and often "fainted" at the end of three minutes. We call it "blackout." In contrast, subjects on Vitamin E could "endure" the experiment for *four* minutes without "much distress." This added stamina with Vitamin E was also corroborated by the pulse rate. For instance, one volunteer's pulse rate, *without* Vitamin E rose, during one three-minute experiment, from 68 to 107; but with Vitamin E, it rose only from

58 to 87. (Vitamin E has the quality of lowering the basic or initial pulse rate in some persons.)

Dr. Goria goes on in a most technical fashion to discuss the various heart "impulses" with and without Vitamin E; interested readers can obtain the original article, of course; but his conclusion is that "Alpha Tocopherol limits the effect of hypoxia on the electrocardiogram." (Aviators, mountain climbers, athletes, deep-sea divers and just so-called average persons, please heed.) Dr. Shute has been trying to interest governmental agencies, official medical groups, and expeditions such as Sir Edmund Hillary's (conqueror of Everest) for years with the proof that Vitamin E in sufficient quantities can reduce the need for oxygen. Let us hope he is eventually successful.

9

The Suppression of Vitamin E

I am told by trusted medical advisors that the story of Vitamin E and its virtual suppression overstrains the credulity of thinking men. Who could believe, for instance, that in our enlightened civilization the orthodox authorities *would* or *could* suppress a treatment for heart disease? *They* also have families, so runs the argument, and they would do anything to save their families as well as themselves.

Alas, the orthodox thinkers have become so stereotyped, so rigid, so fanatic that some members of the group would rather die than consciously admit a wrong of their controlling hierarchy.

In spite of medical and health "scandals" emanating almost every day from Washington and elsewhere, the public cannot believe that a group of policy-making doctors could concertedly act against its interest. Most persons, of course, do not know the history of medicine.

Many are probably unaware that it took some ninety years before orthodox medicine fully accepted the fact that infinitesimal bacteria were responsible for childbed fever or for any other infectious disease. Of course, we know today that many diseases are caused or, at least, are "triggered" by bacteria or viruses. But it is not too widely known, even among doctors, that back in the 1840's, Dr. Ignaz Semmelweiss demonstrated without a doubt that the death rate of new-born infants and their mothers decreased almost to zero when the obstetrician had sterilized his hands. It is hard to believe today that doctors did not realize this need for some form of sterilization, especially when proceeding from the dissecting room to the delivery table. But they didn't, and even after a trial period in which the death rate dropped radically, Semmelweiss' colleagues returned to their old ways, and the infant death rate went back up. Eventually this pioneer of antisepsis in obstetrics died in an institution, insane, after many years of fighting the orthodox medical profession—completely disillusioned with its professed ideals.

In a later part of the same century, it took men of the calibre of Lord Lister, Louis Pasteur, Robert Koch, and many others to convince the orthodox that germs did indeed play a role in the diseases of mankind; you probably did not know, however, that all of these medical pioneers were ridiculed, even lampooned, by their confreres.

Should you question a doctor today about medical history and the fact that he and the society he belongs to have frequently denigrated any truly new or original discovery, he will likely reply: "Ah, but that's a thing of the past. We're scientific now!"

Then you should recommend that he read some books [31] which indicate that we in the twentieth century are, in many respects, just as unscientific as in the past, that the medical oligarchy has seized such control of his mind that he actually believes what he is saying. The propaganda issuing from the formidable headquarters of the American Medical Association in Chicago and the various governmental agencies under the AMA's scientific domination have brainwashed even *his* thinking. But you really cannot blame the individual doctor too much. How is he to know, for instance, that reports on Vitamin E have been squelched or ignored? How is he to know that he is not receiving the truth from what he considers the citadel of medical honesty?

[31] *The Vitamins in Medicine,* Bicknell, Prescott; *Quality Foods for Health,* Chappelle; *Are Doctors Really Inhuman?,* George Bernard Shaw; *Chemicals in Your Food,* Bicknell; *The Doctor Business,* Carter; *Cancer: Disease of Civilization?,* Stefansson.

Doctors are just like other persons in desiring security. They, also, desire to be part of the "In-Group," and they, also, fear to transgress against the Group's laws or regulations. Inexorably those who do are the "bad (unorthodox) boys." The Group reaction: "He shouldn't have been a doctor in the first place, if he's not going to fit into the way we think and the way we do things."

So almost all great medical innovators are "bad boys," who are ridiculed or ignored, often their whole life-time. Quite a few see the "error" of their ways, some after being ejected from their medical societies, relieved of hospital privileges, or ostracized by their associates. Indeed, it takes a very strong man to withstand such treatment in the interest of truth. However, fortunately for the human race, there were, and are, individuals who have withstood such pressures. These are the ones we have to thank for progress.

Official groups depend heavily on the fact that people forget quickly what the AMA, *et al.*, announced yesterday—even if it is proven completely wrong tomorrow, as it happens in innumerable cases. The "error" will be completely forgotten and only the new and "truthful" findings will be remembered.

I am sure that if the AMA reverses its decision concerning Vitamin E, anent heart disease, as a result of intense pressure, its excuse for ignoring and suppressing the evidence as long as possible will be: "We, being scientific, waited until the scientific evidence was absolutely demonstrated. Of course we *now* believe in Vitamin E." It is, indeed, unfortunate that organized groups such as the American Medical Association have so much control over all governmental agencies, as well as those groups who solicit and collect millions of dollars to "fight" various diseases. These powers have managed to gain almost complete control of the views of the government, the press, and the public—having set themselves up as the only "respectable" source of medical information and/or treatment. They will not hesitate to crush opposing views, even if the opposition should come from within their own ranks.

Whatever does not fall within the sphere of the cliques' opinions suffers violent attacks, which pose under the guise of destroying medical "quackery." Unfortunately, these attacks are often launched before the orthodox have even examined the evidence. However, heart and cancer specialists, and specialists of other diseases as well, cannot conceal their delight when a proposed remedy is "discredited" by the orthodox groups to which they belong. It is obvious to anyone who studies the problem of medical practice and research that almost no practicing specialist wants a cure to be found in his particular field. It is only the young, and naive researcher, or the old researcher or clinical practitioner who cannot be harmed by the orthodox poseurs, who will dare to advance unorthodox theories and practices. There is also the occasional researcher or clinical practitioner who will dare to defend what he considers scientific evidence. These latter are usually quickly disposed of by the powers that be, or they will apologize and give up entirely their "misconcepts," or else ostensibly they will abandon their absurd notions and fight "underground."

The Drs. Shute happen to be among those few researcher-clinicians who have refused to be pushed a micrometer measure from the truth of their findings. And they and their followers have suffered from the vengeance wreaked upon them for their brashness in defying the orthodox position. The following serves as a typical example of Medical Orthodoxy in action:

Several hundred patients and ex-patients of the Shute Clinic who had been treated successfully with Vitamin E therapy for cardiovascular conditions, formed what they termed "The Cardiac Society." They wanted to bring the substance which had saved them to the attention of other victims and potential victims of heart disorders.

Among other activities, the Cardiac Society established offices in Detroit. The Society sold the Shutes' popularized version of their book *Alpha Tocopherol [Vitamin E] in Cardiovascular Disease,* which had been directed to the medical profession. The popular version was entitled *Your Heart and*

Vitamin E. The Society seemed well on the way to getting people interested in Vitamin E.

To raise money for their activities and to save people from heart disease, the Society began distributing and selling Vitamin E capsules of the sort which were used in the Shute experiments. This action provided the various federal agencies with the necessary ammunition to destroy the Cardiac Society and the "dangerous propaganda" it was promoting that Vitamin E was of value in heart disease. The AMA, calmly ignoring the mass of evidence, pooh-poohed the idea that Vitamin E could possibly have any effect on heart diseases. It enlisted the federal agencies on its behalf—which was not a difficult task—and disaster befell the Cardiac Society. Before its demolition (and Vitamin E's, to a large degree) was complete, the Orthodoxy even commandeered the services of the U.S. Post Office. Letters addressed to the Society were (and are) returned to the sender marked "Fraudulent." Thus did Authoritarian Medicine show its power to crush anything and anyone daring to present views opposing its own. There were no clever, subtle tactics—just the top executives exerting their influence with the federal agencies to obviate the threat of "competitive" therapies—except that the federal agencies prefer to call their actions "co-operating" with recognized medical authorities to "stamp out quackery."

For this great man, E. V. Shute, and his loyal brother, and the numerous reputable researchers throughout the world who have found immense value in Vitamin E, for them to be, in effect, treated practically as common criminals—"using the mails to defraud"—by the official groups is almost too horrendous for our minds to believe.

However, the fact is that due to various pressures both from within and without the country, *eventually* our medical research will bumble and stumble along until finally cancer, heart disease, and other major killers will be conquered—moving at the pace set by the orthodox. We should not let the doctors in control—the politically ambitious, the money-hungry, or the jealous researchers—dictate medical policy and thought. If we continue to follow this policy, the so-called healthiest nation in the world, with 74,000,000 of the 183,000,000 population having one or more chronic diseases, will have even fewer healthy individuals in the future.

Our civilization is so enlightened, we are told constantly, that we have no need to worry in any field of human endeavor. Yet the medical student is indoctrinated quite early. He is taught that the doctor's profession is sacrosanct; therefore, it has a right to do anything it pleases. The incipient doctor is also taught that he himself is inviolable, as long as he memorizes the textbooks and absorbs his teachers' thinking. A "good" doctor learns quickly enough that, by virtue of treating the illnesses of human beings, he represents the power of life or death over the individual. However, in order to perpetuate that power, he must maintain and foster the edicts of the organized medical groups no matter what they may be.

With this type of authoritarian education pounded into him day after day, year after year, who can blame the average physician for being brainwashed, so that in time he comes to really believe what he is told? For the few mavericks who still try to practice unorthodox medicine after their indoctrination, retaliation is usually swift. It often begins as a whispering campaign and ends—if the recreant does not "swing into line"— with loss of hospital privileges or even open censure and/or ouster from the medical society. The latter usually proves disastrous to a physician attempting to earn a living. Usually, however, even the "worst" of the "original" thinkers come back to the fold before it is too late.

We do not mean to imply that every doctor who is censured or ousted is an original thinker or a great scientist, far ahead of his time. There *are* quacks, unfortunately, in the medical profession. There are doctors who deliberately establish a medical racket in the form of unnecessary operations, for instance, and those who, preying on the gullibility of the uninformed, will charge exorbitant fees for "cures" and nostrums, which they, themselves, know to be worthless. And there are doctors who are capable of falsifying reports on a beneficial treatment —which they *know* to be beneficial—in order to gain commercial rights to the substance, later planning to announce that the substance is indeed beneficial.

Very fortunately, these reprehensible activities in the medical profession are rare. The rank and file M.D., due to his authoritarian education, cannot conceive of the hierarchy doing any wrong in the *crooked* sense; therefore he shuts off his mind to any such nonsense. However, once you can force him, with facts, to reopen his mind, as for example, to the action of Vitamin E on heart disease, his response is usually one of overwhelmed amazement. Then, depending on his real desire to search for the truth, he will either try the proposed agent (but please keep my name secret!) or else reject it completely.

Even when a doctor finds that the agent is effective, he may still shy away from such treatment until it has been "accepted." After all, can *you* blame him? How would *you* react to ostracism by your friends and to the probable loss of all income?

No one, today, questions Vitamin E's chemical identity or the need for it in the body. The authorities do question, however, its usefulness in the prevention and treatment of many so-called degenerative diseases. It is obvious that these authorities have not read the world literature or else have chosen to ignore it. And how can you explain the fact that many doctors in Canada are using it privately for themselves and their close relatives and yet are afraid to prescribe it for their patients?

The real breakthrough in the history of Vitamin E will come when both the authorities and practicing physicians have examined all the evidence, and feel free to prescribe Vitamin E. Researchers will then be granted adequate sums of money to investigate the substance thoroughly and to prove to the public once and for all the importance of Vitamin E for our general health and especially for the heart.

Appendix A

The Current Status of Alpha Tocopherol in Cardiovascular Disease[*]

By Evan Shute, B.A., M.B., F.R.C.S.(C)
The Shute Institute
London, Canada

ALPHA TOCOPHEROL ONLY

Let us make clear initially that we use the term vitamin E (when we do use it) merely because it has long been recognized by the medical profession, because it is popular medical slang, and because the laity recognize it as an entity. It is not an entity, of course, but a mixture of seven tocopherols. These should be referred to individually by accurate writers, just as we refer nowadays not to vitamin B but to its components; e.g., thiamin, riboflavin, pantothenic acid, pyridoxene, or niacin. *We* always mean alpha tocopherol when we speak of vitamin E, just as most scientific writers do. The distinction still seems to need emphasis.

THE BASIC PROPERTIES OF ALPHA TOCOPHEROL SUGGESTING ITS USE IN CARDIOVASCULAR DISEASE

In proper dosage, alpha tocopherol is therapeutically effective in the treatment of cardiovascular disease. We have not said

[*] Reprinted from *The Summary*, December, 1959.

131

"for any person so afflicted," although this may be true. Possible exceptions are an acute arterial embolism, or a tremendous gangrene which even operation might not save, or any moribund patient, or the severest haemorrhage, or a huge aneurysm, or a wound of the heart or great vessels. Even in such cases it never could be argued that tocopherol had *nothing* to offer, because of its extraordinarily diverse physiological and biochemical properties.

What properties make it useful in treating cardiovascular diseases?

(a) *It resembles digitalis in its action on the hypoxic heart.* Digitalis is *the* classical heart drug, used almost universally in almost every type of heart disease except the congenital types. The evidence for its similarity to digitalis appears in:

Govier, W. M., Yanz, N., and Grelis, M. E. (U.S.A.): *J. Pharmacol. & Exp. Ther.*, 88:373, 1946.
Spaulding, M. E., and Graham, W. D. (Canada): *J.B.C.*, 170:711, 1947.

This alone would establish alpha tocopherol as a useful heart drug. In fact, such functional similarity to digitalis would make that *difficult* to deny.

(b) *It is uniquely able to improve tissue oxygenation.* Oxygen deficit is characteristic of almost all heart disease, certainly cases in failure, and even in the earliest phases. No other physiological substance has this property to anything like the same degree:

Hove, E. L., Hickman, K. C. D., and Harris, P. L. (U.S.A.): *Arch. Biochem.*, 8:395, 1945.
Zierler, K. L., Folk, B. P., Eyzaguirre, C., Jarcho, L. W., Grob, D., and Lilienthal, J. L. (U.S.A.): Second Vitamin Symposium, New York, 1949.
Vaccari, F. (Italy): *Cuore e Circolazione*, 35:164, 173, 1951.
Hummel, J. P., and Melville, R. S. (U.S.A.): *J. Biol. Chem.*, 101:383, 1951.

Goria, I. R. (Italy): *Boll. della Soc. Ital. di Biol. Sper.*, **29**:1275, 1953.

Telford, I. R., Wiswell, O. B., Smith, E. L., Clark, R. T., Jr., Tomaschefski, J. F., and Criscuolo, D. (U.S.A.): Air University School of Aviation Medicine, Project No. 21-1201-0013, Report #4, May, 1954 (Randolph Field, Texas).

Telford, I. R., Wiswell, O. B., and Smith, E. L. (U.S.A.): *Proc. Soc. Exp. Biol. & Med.*, **87**:162, 1954.

Frey, J. (Germany): *Arch. f. exp. Path. u. Pharmakol.*, **221**:456, 1954.

Saha, H. (India): *J. Indian Med. Assoc.*, **23**:428, 1954.

Horvath, G., Kowacsovics, T., and Potendy, A. (Hungary): *Acta Physiol. Hung.*, E-suppl. 41, 1956.

Scapinelli, G. E. (Italy): *Sperimentale*, **106**:374, 1956.

This alone would establish alpha tocopherol as *indispensable* in nearly all heart and vascular disease. This is impossible to deny. To make matters even clearer, Nason et al. have implicated tocopherol as "one of the active components of the terminal respirating chain in mammalian skeletal and heart muscle tissue." It appears to be a co-factor in the cytochrome C system.

Nason, A., Donaldson, K. O., and Lehman, I. R. (U.S.A.): *Trans. N.Y. Acad. Sci.*, **20**:27, 1957.

(c) *Alpha tocopherol has been described by at least two first-rate groups as an antithrombin:*

Zierler, K. L., Grob, D., and Lilienthal, J. L. (U.S.A.): *Am. J. Physiol.*, **153**:127, 1948.

Kay, J. H., Hutton, S. B., Weiss, G. N., and Ochsner, A. (U.S.A.): *Surgery*, **28**:124, 1950.

By others it has been said to influence clotting time, thrombokinase, even the vascular endothelium. Indeed, one well-known Italian worker said at the Venice Congress of 1955 that vitamin E should henceforth be called the "angiophilic" vitamin, referring to its ability to protect blood vessels. Some of the relevant papers are:

Jesson, K. E., Glavind, J., Hartmann, S., and Dam, N. (Denmark): *Acta Path.*, **29**:73, 1951.

Constantini, A., and Ricci, C. (Italy): *Le Chirurgie Gen.*, 1:300, 1951.

Masure, R., and Van Ruyssevelt, J. (Belgium): *Rev. Belg. Path. Med. exp.*, 22:73, 1952.

Heymann, A., and Stamm, O. (Switzerland): *Gynaecologia*, 140:224, 1955.

Galletti, F., Gelli, G., and Giungi, F. (Italy): *Acta Vitaminol.*, 9:71, 1955.

Mazzetti, G. M. (Italy): *Acta Vitaminol.*, 10:213, 1956.

Whatever the mechanism by which it acts on intravascular clots already formed, its effect in resolving such thrombosis has been attested by many first-rate observers. For example:

Castagna, R., and Impallomeni, G. (Italy): *Biol. Soc. Piemont Chir.*, 18:155, 1948.

de Oliviera, D. (Brazil): *Separata de O Hospital*, 36:135, 1949.

Boyd, A. M., Ratcliffe, A. H., James, G. W. H., and Jepson, R. P. (England): *Lancet*, 2:132, 1949.

Mantero, O., Rindi, B., and Trozzi, L. (Italy): *Atti. Cong. Cardiologia*, Stresa, May, 1949.

Sturup, H. (Norway): *Nordisk Medicin*, 43:721, 1950.

Ochsner, A., Kay, J. H., deCamp, P. T., Hutton, S. B., and Balla, G. A. (U.S.A.): *Ann. Surg.*, 131:652, 1950.

Ochsner, A., De Bakey, M. E., and deCamp, P. T. (U.S.A.): *J.A.M.A.*, 144:831, 1950.

Ochsner, A. (U.S.A.): *Postgrad. Med.*, 10:794, 1951.

Ged (France): Medical Thesis, Sim, Paris, 1951, No. 471.

Bauer, R. (U.S.A.): *Wien. klin. Woch.*, 31:552, 1951.

Reifferscheid, M., and Matis, P. (Germany): *Med. Welt.*, 20:1168, 1951.

Crump, W. E., and Heiskell, E. F. (U.S.A.): *Texas State J. of Med.*, 48:11, 1952.

Terrel Speed (U.S.A.): Abstract of Discussion, *Texas State J. of Med.*, 48:11, 1952.

Schmid, S. (Austria): *Wien. klin. Woch.*, 64:128, 1952.

Wagner, H. (Germany): *Aertszliche Woch.*, 7:248, 1952.

Krieg, E. (Germany): Book pub. by Urban and Schwarzenberg, Munich, 1952.

Dominguez, J. P., and Dominguez, R. (Spain): *Angiologia*, 5:51, 1953.

Kraus, H. H. (Germany): *Zent. f. Gyn.*, 75:1249, 1953.

Schiavina, G. P. (Italy): *Policlinico*, 61:581, 1954.

Vitak, B. (Czechoslovakia): *Ceskoslovenska Gynaekologie,* 19:345, 1954.

Wilson, M. G., and Parry, E. W. (England): *Lancet,* 1:486, 1954.

Vecchietti, G. (Italy): Proc. 3rd Internat. Cong. on Vit. E, Venice, Italy, September 1955, p. 209.

Bruchnerova, O. (Czechoslovakia): *Unitrni Ickarstvi,* 1:137, 1955.

Aghina, A., and Cerra, R. (Italy): *Gazz. Int. Med. Clin.,* 7:444, 1955.

Suffel, P. (Canada): *Can. M.A.J.,* 74:715, 1956.

Szirmai, E. (Hungary): Personal communication—*Summary,* 10:87, 1958.

Moreover, some of these workers have remarked on its unique values in preventing embolism, in which it is so much more effective than its rival anticoagulants. For example:

Crump, W. E., and Heiskell, E. F. (U.S.A.): *Texas State J. of M.,* 48:11, 1952.

Wilson, M. G., and Parry, E. W. (England): *Lancet,* 1:486, 1954.

Suffel, P. (Canada): *Can. M.A.J.,* 74:715, 1956.

Blood clotting is always blood clotting, whether in a leg or the brain, in a vein or an artery, and must always occur by identical mechanisms above or below the diaphragm. That is the reasoning behind the widespread use of the anticoagulants, first made available for leg and other peripheral venous clots, in coronary artery disease. The line of reasoning making dicumarol useful in coronary disease automatically makes alpha tocopherol more useful still, and, of course, it is infinitely safer.

Now, since clotting is one of the major hazards in most cardiovascular disease, whether coronary thrombosis or cerebral thrombosis, auricular fibrillation, hypertensive or atherosclerotic heart disease, or diabetic atherosclerosis, and so on, the prompt lysis of clot or prevention of clotting recurrence or of embolism is a vital factor in its management. No one can deny this. The safety factor here, the fact that alpha tocopherol *never* induces haemorrhage as the rival anticoagulants so regularly do, that it needs no weekly prothrombin or other difficult laboratory tests to ensure only a comparative safety, that it is safe, cheap and readily administered by any physician, not only by specialists, renders it the drug of choice in any situation calling for an anti-coagulant, unless, just *possibly,* it be an acute arterial thrombosis. Moreover, it cannot worsen a cerebral haemorrhage, as anti-coagulants must do frequently, and it is recently becoming clear that such haemorrhage, as distinct from cerebral thrombosis, can be difficult to recognize.

Should it be pointed out that we led in this field?—*Ann. Kansas City Acad. Med.,* 1946–47–47, p. 47.

(d) *The action of vitamin E upon scar is unique, although somewhat inconstant.* No other substance has even been found which can both "melt away" or soften existing scar, even of many years' duration, and can prevent such scar formation as is always encountered in wounds or burns not treated by alpha tocopherol; namely, scar that contracts as it heals. It is scarcely necessary to point out how important this property can be for many cases of chronic rheumatic heart disease where the myocardium is full of tiny scarred areas and the valves are often deformed by scar tissue. It could be of interest in the scars induced by coronary athero-sclerosis, hypertensive heart disease, and so forth. Why must doctors always treat old heart scars by such dangerous and often ineffective means as those of surgery? Is it not a great step forward to think of preventing valve scars and resolving them medically?

Suitable references are numerous. All stem from the pioneer studies of C. L. Steinberg of Rochester and need scarcely be cited here because so widely known:

Steinberg, C. L. (U.S.A.): *Med. Clin. N. Amer.,* **30**:22, 1946; *Ann. N.Y. Acad. Sci.,* **52**:380, 1949.

Scardino, P. L., and Hudson, P. B. (U.S.A.): *Proc. 2nd Vit. E Conf.,* New York, 1949.

Scardino, P. L., and Scott, W. W. (U.S.A.): *Ann. N.Y. Acad. Sci.,* **52**:390, 1949.

Cortesi, C. (Italy): *Boll. della Malattie Dell'Orecchio, Della Gola, Del Naso,* **68**:343, 1950.

Heinsen, H. A., and Koker, H. (Germany): *Deutsche med. Woch.,* **76**:887, 1951.

Van Duzen, R. E., and Mustain, R. (U.S.A.): *J. Urol.,* **65**:1033, 1951.

Steinberg, C. L. (U.S.A.): *Arch. Surg.,* **63**:824, 1951.

Edgerton, M. T., Jr., Hanrahan, E. M., and Davis, W. B. (U.S.A.): *Plastic & Reconstructive Surg.,* **8**:224, 1951.

Nikolowski, W. (Germany): *Strahlentherapie,* **87**:113, 1952.

Gibson, H. R. B. (England): *Brit. Med. J.,* **2**:446, 1952.

Ross, J. A. (England): *Ibid.,* **2**:232, 1952.

Blaxter, K. L., and Wood, W. A. (Scotland): *B.J. Nutrit.,* **6**:144, 1952.

Piana, C. (Italy): *Acta Vitaminol.,* **6**:69, 1952.

Kirk, J. E., and Chieffi, M. (U.S.A.): *Proc. Soc. Exper. Biol. & Med.,* **80**:565, 1952.

Waller, J. X., and Breese, W. C. (U.S.A.): *J. Urol.,* **68**:623, 1952.

Aurig, G., and Susse, H. J. (Germany): *Strahlentherapie,* **89**:433, 1952.

Ruggiero, A., and Sabbatini, C. (Italy): *Gior. Ital. di Chir.,* **8**:506, 1952.

de Mello, A. (Spain): *Arquiv. Mineiros de Leprologia,* **11**:148, 1952.

Lohel, H. (Germany): *Deutsche Gesundheitswesen,* **7**:1365, 1952.

Dahl, O. (Sweden): *Nord. Med.,* **50**:969, 1953.

Gartmann, H., and Sierler, H. (Germany): *Derm. Woch.,* **128**:1213, 1953.

Pult, H. (Germany): *Deutsche med. Woch.,* **79**:471, 1954.

This unique property of vitamin E alone would render it a drug of choice in many a cardiovascular problem. Remember, too, that no other substance has this property.

The prevention of scar formation is graphically demonstrated by photographs in our possession, one of them showing a second-degree burn over the knuckles of a hand, the hand showing *perfect flexion when healed*. This result is unbelievable, but has been duplicated in other patients, and these patients have been shown to medical groups for their careful scrutiny.

No other substance possesses either of these abilities—another example of the unrivalled therapeutic powers of vitamin E. Here is a result alpha tocopherol produces which is quite unexplainable by present pathological knowledge, and yet has been proven by many medical observers all over the world. This illustrates how dangerous it can be to decide *a priori* what alpha tocopherol can or cannot do.

(e) *Vitamin E appears to be a muscle stimulant per se.* This action of vitamin E on muscle in the intact animal or in man has long been difficult to make sure of because such benefits could also accrue due to increased oxygen utilization by muscle or to improved circulation in muscle, as has been suggested above. However, recent studies on *isolated* muscles have proven it to have specific effects here:

Corsi, A., and Margreth, A. (Italy): *Sperimentale,* 107:415, 1957.
Schottelius, B. A., and Schottelius, D. D. (U.S.A.): *Am. J. Physiol.,* 193:219, 1958.

and go far to explain the early studies of Percival, Curto, and others.

Vaccari, for example, showed that vitamin E had a favourable effect on both coronary flow and the muscular contractility of the heart of frogs. Indeed, the isolated heart perfused with alpha tocopherol survived 126 minutes, as opposed to 75 minutes for his controls, presumably due to an additive effect of both these properties of alpha tocopherol.

This effect on muscle alone would justify the use of alpha tocopherol in almost every cardiac disability, where either a primarily damaged myocardium or a myocardium secondarily impaired by congenital defects of the great vessels or septa or by endocardial inflammations and their valvular sequelae, or where one should support a myocardium which, labouring against increased peripheral resistance in either the greater or lesser circulation, or against congestion, has begun to weaken. No other tonic substance can be suggested, unless digitalis has some value here.

(f) *Vitamin E improves the capillary wall that has become impaired by one mechanism or another.* Here its only rival is rutin—perhaps. There is a good deal of evidence on this, adduced by such workers as:

Mason, K. E. (U.S.A.): *Yale J. Biol. & Med.,* **14**:605, 1942.

Minkowski, A. (France): *Arch. Franc. de Pediatrie,* **6**:276, 1949.

Comi, G., and Nesi, G. (Italy): *Riv. Crit. de Clin. Med.,* **50**:214, 1950.

Ames, S. R., Baxter, J. G., and Griffith, J. G. (U.S.A.): *Internat. Rev. of Vit. Res.,* **22**:401, 1951.

Serafini, U. M., and Pratesi, G. (Italy): *Boll. Soc. Ital. Biol. Sper.,* **27**:1660, 1951.

Coselli, F. (Italy): *Boll. D'Oculista,* **31**:271, 1952.

Funfak, H. (Germany): *Artzl. Forsch.,* **6**:247, 1952.

ten Berge, B. G., and Polak, R. (Holland): First World Cong. on Fertility and Sterility, New York, May, 1953.

Prosperi, P., and Dell'Orso, S. (Italy): *Riv. di Clin. Pediat.,* **52**:501, 1953.

Dotti, F., and Leoni, R. (Italy): *Gior. di Clin. Med.,* **35**:179, 1954.

We first reported this observation in *Science,* **103**:762, 1946 and *Urol. & Cut. Rev.,* **50**:732, 1946.

Were it only for this property, vitamin E would have a place in the pharmacopoeia of every scientific cardiologist who is aware that inflammatory and degenerative processes damage capillary walls, produce damaging local or more general oedemas and exudates, and that these may go on to overwhelm and drown his patient as the circulatory mechanism destroys itself by constant leakage.

(g) *At the moment, vast sums of research money are being spent on, and many teams of research workers are engaged in, studies of the process of atherosclerosis,* regarded in the United States generally as the most significant factor in the causation of degenerative cardiovascular disease. Partly this is directed at cholesterol metabolism generally and partly at atherosclerotic animals in an effort to produce humanlike lesions and their resolution or prevention.

The evidence as to whether vitamin E influences cholesterol metabolism is conflicting (*J.A.M.A.,* **140**:768, 1949). In huge doses it almost certainly does (Greenblatt, et al.: *Proc. Am. Soc. Study Arteriosclerosis,* **16**:508, 1957). But we wish to point up a more direct approach, that of Weitzel, et al. It is well known that hens as they age tend to develop an atherosclerosis like that of man. This can be prevented or halted by the combination of vitamins A and E, either alone being relatively ineffective.

The pertinent references are:

Weitzel, G., Schon, H., and Gey, F. (Germany): *Klin. Woch.,* **33**:772, 1955.
Weitzel, G., Schon, H., Gey, F., and Buddecke, E. (Germany): *Z. Physiol. Chem., Hoppe-Seyler's,* **304**:247, 1956.
Kern, H., Meissner, O., and Spies, R. (Austria): *Wien. med. Woch.,* **108**:175, 1958.
Guillemin, P. (France): *Rev. de Praticien,* 8:1662, 1958.

This observation alone would make any cardiovascular expert feel that vitamin E had a major role to play in his specialty. We suspect that this observation short-cuts the vast sums being expended on sitosterols, nicotinic acid, diets low in dairy products. Indeed, it might even rehabilitate the dairy industry which has lost so much face over animal fats in the current cholesterol purge.

We first called attention to the value of alpha tocopherol in the *complications* of atherosclerosis in *Surg., Gyn., & Obst.,* **86**:1, 1948.

The prognosis for survival in intermittent claudication has recently been shown to be much reduced. Tolgyes, however, when considering patients treated with alpha tocopherol, found the prognosis greatly improved over comparable figures in the literature. This bears upon the effect of alpha tocopherol on the ominous atherosclerotic process:

Tolgyes, S. (Canada): *Summary,* **11**:9, 1959.

The direct, controlled studies on intermittent claudication carried out by Jones and Livingstone (*Lancet,* **2**:602, 1958) have a bearing here. Admittedly, peripheral arteriosclerosis has anatomical peculiarities not shared by the coronary system, and vice versa, but fundamentally the atherosclerotic process in one artery is like that in another. Here is an example of the atherosclerosis which obstructs great leg arteries sufficiently to produce muscle anoxaemia and cramp, relieved effectively by alpha tocopherol. Can anyone deny the strong case this makes for the use of the same substance to relieve heart muscle pain produced by the same type of arterial obstruction and hypoxia?

(h) *Vitamin E is occasionally a diuretic, a fact which is of importance in managing every failing heart.* This action has been corroborated by others:

Heinson, H. A., and Koker, H. (Germany): *Deutsche med. Woch.,* **76**:487, 1951.

Krohn, B. G., and Pottinger, F. M. (U.S.A.): *Ann. West. Med. & Surg.,* **6**:484, 1952.

Becker-Freyseng, H. (Germany): *Arch. f. exp. Path. u. Pharmak.,* **214**:411, 1952.

Frey, J. (Germany): *Arch. f. exp. Path. u. Pharmak.,* **221**:466, 1954.

Our first observations here were in:

Vogelsang, A., Shute, E. V., and Shute, W. E.: *Med. Rec.,* **160**:1, 1947.

(i) *Occasionally vitamin E is hypotensive,* which is a helpful factor in the management of many a cardiovascular patient. This observation rests on our own studies and those of such workers as:

Pescetti, G. (Italy): *Arch. e Maragliani di Patol. e Clin.,* **6**:325, 1951.

Allardyce, J., Salter, J., and Rixon, R. (Canada): *Am. J. Physiol.,* **164**:48, 1951.

Glauner, W. (Germany): *Deutsche med. Woch.,* **77**:627, 1952.

Holtkamp, W. (Germany): *Zent. f. Gyn.,* **75**:1099, 1953.

O'Connor, V. R., and Hodges, J. P. S. (England): Third Internat. Cong. on Vit. E, Venice, Italy, 1955.

Kern, H., Meissner, O., and Spies, R. (Austria): *Wien. med. Woch.,* **108**:175, 1958.

This fact alone would make vitamin E valuable in a great fraction of all cardiovascular problems. High blood pressure is a very grave complication in so many patients.

He would be a brave man, or a reckless or an ignorant man, who would deny that an agent so versatile, so potent, so unique, would not be of value in treating every type of cardiovascular disease known, with the *possible* exception of some rare types listed earlier in this discussion. Even there it probably has something to offer.

Cardiovascular disease is one unit. What applies in one part of the circulation applies in another, with the relatively few exceptions dependent on local anatomical peculiarities or unknown racial factors. Hence the justification for calling the great journal dealing principally with heart disease by such a name as *Circulation*. Hence the extension of the use of anticoagulants to coronary and cerebral vascular disease. Hence our extension to heart diseases of the vascular uses of alpha tocopherol which have been so widely confirmed.

Many, many workers all over the world, as if by a common conspiracy, have lent support to the contention that alpha tocopherol is valuable in the treatment of heart disease. We list them here:

Santacroce, A. (Italy): *Policlinico* (sezione practica), **48**:2119, 1942.

Butturini, U. (Italy): *Gior. di Clin. Med.*, **27**:400, 1946.

Govier, W. M., Yanz, N., and Grelis, M. E. (U.S.A.): *J. Pharmacol. & Exp. Ther.*, **88**:373, 1946.

Molotchik, M. B. (U.S.A.): *Med. Rec.*, **160**:667, 1947.

Lambert, N. H. (Eire): *Vet. Rec.*, **27**:355, 1947.

Pin, L. (France): Thesis, M. Lavergne, Paris, 1947.

Spaulding, M. E., and Graham, W. D. (Canada): *J.B.C.*, **170**:711, 1947.

Agadjaniantz, N. (France): *J. de Med. de Paris*, **68**:29, 48, 105, 229, 1948.

Gram, C. N. J., and Schmidt, V. (Denmark): *Nordisk Med.*, **37**:82, 1948.

Ramos, H. (Brazil): *Publ. Medicas São Paulo*, **25**, 177, **67**, 1948.

Valatz, A. (France): *Toulouse Med.*, **48**:275, 1948.

Dedichen, J. (Norway): *Nord. Med.*, 41:324, 1949.

Galeone, A. (Italy): *Rec. Prog. Med.*, 7:238, 1949.

Mantero, O., Rindi, B., and Trozzi, L. (Italy): *Atti. Cong. Cardiologia,* Stresa, May, 1949.

Steinberg, C. L. (U.S.A.): *Ann. N.Y. Acad. Sci.*, 52:380, 1949.

Galeone, A., and Minelli, M. (Italy): *Minerva Med.*, 46:694, 1950.

Mantero, O. (Italy): *L'Ospedale Maggiore*, 38:638, 1950.

Freire, S. A. (Brazil): *Rev. de Gyn. e d'Obst.*, 44:19, 1950.

Scardigli, G., Mininni, G., and Capelli, P. (Italy): *La Riforma Med.*, 64:895, 1950.

Baguena, H. (Spain): *Rev. Med. de Liege*, 5:622, 1950.

Schmidt, L. (England): *Med. World*, 72:296, 1950.

O'Connor, V. R. (England): *Ibid.*, 72:299, 1950.

Pendl, F. (Germany): *Deut. med. Wochschr.*, 75:1405, 1950.

Anson, P. J. (Germany): *Landarzt*, 26:262, 1950.

Seidenari, R., Mars, G., and Morpurgo, M. (Italy): *Acta Gerontol.*, 1:55, 1951.

Vaccari, F. (Italy): *Cuore e Circulazione*, 35:164, 1951.

Vaccari, F. (Italy): *Ibid.*, 35:173, 1951.

Mouquin, M. (France): *Rev. du Practicien*, 1:479, 1951.

Terzani, G. (Italy): *Policlinica-Sezione Prat.*, 58:1381, 1951.

Coatsworth, R. C. (Canada): *Summary*, 3:25, 1951.

Khastgir, A. R. (England): *Summary*, 4:6, 1952.

Seliger, H. (Germany): *Deutsche Med.*, 3:20, 1952.

Schmid, S. (Austria): *Wien. klin. Woch.*, 64:128, 1952.

Goria, A., and Mallen, J. (Italy): *Boll. della Soc. Ital. di Biol. Sper.*, 29:1278, 1953.

Merucci, P., and Gilot, G. B. (Italy): *Arch. de Vecchi per l'Anat. Patol. e la Med. Clin.*, 19:737, 1953.

Gibbons, A. J., Howes, B. G., and Smits, E. (U.S.A.): *Am. Heart J.*, 45:122, 1953.

Preziosi, P. (Italy): *Riforma Med.*, 67:212, 1953.

Leone, A., and Sulis, E. (Italy): *Ann. Ital. Pediat.*, 6:1, 1953.

Beckman, R., and Kuhlmann, F. (Germany): *Munch. med. Woch.*, 96:970, 1954.

Pult, H. (Germany): *Deutsche med. Woch.*, 79:471, 1954.

Hillman, R. W., Nerb, L., and Hutz, H. (U.S.A.): *N.Y. State J. of Med.*, 55:2787, 1955.

Puente-Dominguez, J. L., and Domingues, P. (Spain): *Rev. Española de Cardiologia*, 9:30, 1955.

O'Connor, V. R., and Hodges, J. P. S. (England): *Proc. 3rd Internat. Cong. Vit. E*, Venice, 1955, p. 454.

Lambert, N. H. (Ireland): *Ibid.*, p. 610.

Bouman, J., and Slater, E. C. (Holland): *Nature,* 177:1281, 1956.
Meyer, E., Jutting, G., and Schmidt, S. (Germany): *Munch. med. Woch.,* 98:202, 1956.
Diaz, F. V. (?): *Progr. y Clin.,* 3:351, 1956.
Aslan, A. (Roumania): *Med. Klin.,* 52:1758, 1957.
Guillemin, P. (France): *Rev. du Practicien,* 8:1662, 1958.

Could so many workers in so many different countries have entered into collusion to support this suggestion of ours, now 13 years old? [As of 1959.—*Ed.*]

We should call attention to just a few specific reports, perhaps. Lambert, the great Dublin veterinarian, has put dogs in heart failure back into the hunting field on vitamin E therapy! Here is the best possible demonstration of the value of alpha tocopherol in restoring heart muscle and improving tissue oxygenation and circulation in dogs panting for breath beside the hearth, completely unable to chase any hare or fox, and completely inaccessible to "suggestion" by a doctor. It is equivalent to putting a man in hospital in heart failure back in a mile race beside youngsters. This single observation, widely corroborated amongst dog lovers everywhere, would demonstrate the unique values of alpha tocopherol in cardiovascular disease.

Power and Kosmal have reviewed a large series of heart patients treated with alpha tocopherol, the former studying left bundle branch block and the latter coronary occlusions. Both showed figures at least as good as those published for the classical modes of treatment, with large fractions of their patients still alive and therefore bound to improve the data greatly with the passage of further time. These are two groups of highly prejudiced cardiac patients, in whom survival is a crucial criterion:

Power, P. (Canada): *Summary,* 10:49, 1958.
Kosmal, R. (Canada): *Ibid.,* 11:5, 1959.

There is a long list of workers who have found that depriving animals of alpha tocopherol sooner or later induces focal myocardial lesions. The unanimity of these findings is striking, the lesions are numerous and important, nine species are involved, and, although it is questionable that the human heart presents focal lesions similar to those seen in most tocopherol-deficient animals, the perivascular lesions in the myocardium found in alpha tocopherol-deficient calves are not too unlike the Aschoff nodules found in rheumatic human heart muscles. The electrocardiographic changes seen in association with these myocardial lesions in experimental animals are analogous to those seen in damaged human hearts. The picture is definitely one of alpha tocopherol deficiency regularly producing myocardial damage. Should only the human heart be able to escape the corresponding results of nearly comparable and certainly *much* more prolonged deficiency of alpha tocopherol? What are the infarcts that have no origin in coronary occlusion (16 to 59 per cent of the total)?:

Madsen, L. L. (U.S.A.): *J. Nutrit.*, 11:471, 1936.

Bird, H. R., and Culton, T. G. (U.S.A.): *Proc. Soc. Exp. Biol. & Med.*, 44:543, 1940.

Houchin, O. B., and Smith, H. W. (U.S.A.): *Am. J. Physiol.*, 141:242, 1941.

Houchin, O. B., and Mattill, H. A. (U.S.A.): *Proc. Soc. Exp. Biol. & Med.*, 50:216, 1942.

Freire, S. A., and Figueiredo, M. B. (Brazil): *Rev. Brazil Biol.*, 3:91, 1943.

Mason, K. E., and Emmel, Y. L. (U.S.A.): *Anat. Rec.*, 92:33, 1945.

Gullickson, T. W., and Calverley, C. E. (U.S.A.): *Science,* 104:312, 1946

Willman, S. P., Loosli, J. K., Asdell, S. A., Morrison, F. B., and Olafson, P. (U.S.A.): *Cornell Veterinarian,* 36:200, 1946.

Gatz, A. J., and Houchin, O. B. (U.S.A.): *Anat. Rec.*, 97:337, 1946.

Martin, G. V., and Faust, F. B. (U.S.A.): *Exp. Med. & Surg.*, 5:405, 1947.

Mason, K. E., and Telford, I. R. (U.S.A.): *Arch. Path.*, 43:363, 1947.

Ruppel, W. (Germany): *Arch. f. Exp. Path. u. Pharmakol.*, 206:584, 1949.

Bragdon, J. H., and Levine, H. D. (U.S.A.): *Am. J. Path.*, 25:265, 1949.

Filer, L. J., Jr., Rumery, R. E., Yu, N. G., and Mason, K. E. (U.S.A.): *Ann. N.Y. Acad. Sci,* 52:284, 1949.

Tunicliffe, E. A. (U.S.A.): Personal Communication, 1949.

146 ALPHA TOCOPHEROL IN CARDIOVASCULAR DISEASE

Blaxter, K. L., Watts, P. S., and Wood, W. A. (Scotland): *Brit. J. Nutrit.*, 5:42, 1951.

Culik, R., Bacigalupo, F. A., Thorp, F., Luecke, R. W., and Nelson, R. H. (U.S.A.): *J. Animal Sci.*, 10:1006, 1951.

Draper, H. H., James, M. F., and Johnson, B. C. (U.S.A.): *J. Nutrit.*, 47:583, 1952.

Blaxter, K. L., Watts, P. S., and Wood, W. A. (Scotland): *Brit. J. Nutrit.*, 6:125, 1952.

Houle, G. R. (U.S.A.): *J. Am. Vet. Med. Assoc.*, 121:485, 1952.

Menschik, Z. (Canada): *Proc. Can. Phys. Soc.*, Quebec Meeting, October 4, 1952.

Bacigalupo, F. A., Alfredson, B. V., Luecke, R. W., and Thorp, F., Jr. (U.S.A.): *Am. J. Vet. Res.*, 14:214, 1953.

Chiung Puh-Lee (U.S.A.): Doctoral Dissertation, U. of Minn., 1953.

Sturkie, P. B., Singsen, E. P., Matterson, L. D., Kazeff, A., and Jungherr, E. L. (U.S.A.): *Am. J. Vet. Res.*, 15:457, 1954.

Sharman, G. A. M. (Scotland): *Vet. Rec.*, 66:275, 1954.

Mulder, A. G., Gatz, A. J., and Tigerman, B. (U.S.A.): *Am. J. Physiol.*, 179:246, 1954.

Frey, J. (Germany): *Arch. f. exp. Path. u. Pharmak.*, 221:466, 1954.

Menschik, Z. (Canada): *Proc. Third Internat. Cong. on Vit. E*, Venice, Italy, September, 1955.

Williams, W. L., and Aronsohn, R. B. (U.S.A.): *Yale J. Biol. & Med.*, 28:515, 1956.

Williams, W. L. (U.S.A.): *Circulation*, 16:952, 1957.

Forbes, R. M., and Draper, H. H. (U.S.A.): *J. Nutrit.*, 65:535, 1958.

But the most important and direct approach to this problem in experimental study has been the work of the Dominguez team on coronary ligation in dogs. These workers produced myocardial infarcts in dogs by tieing the coronary artery, then gave alpha tocopherol to some of them. The results were spectacular. An intense proliferation of new collateral arterial channels entered the infarct area in an effort to heal it. This must be what happens when a man with coronary infarction is given alpha tocopherol. This single experiment corroborates our whole position on the tocopherol management of coronary artery disease.

ALPHA TOCOPHEROL AS A CARDIOVASCULAR PROPHYLACTIC

Now for the idea that vitamin E will prevent heart disease. We have never stated that it would prevent all types of heart disease, nor all cases of any type of heart disease. We have pointed out, however, its *value or power in the prevention of many types of heart disease*. Power is a relative word. It can be 10 per cent effective or 90 per cent. We speak of Great Powers and Small Powers among nations. We descant on the power of insulin to control diabetes, although not all cases are controlled and a 10-unit dose is powerless in a 20-unit case, or a dose at breakfast may be powerless to control the blood sugar all day. Power is always a relative term, because the powers of any drug fail in a recalcitrant patient, or if incorrectly known or used. The wrestler who loses still has power. A rocket at Cape Canaveral has awesome power although it may fall far short of a moon-strike. The anticoagulants are so named for their power to prevent blood clotting, yet often fail to do so, even with proper prothrombin regulation (for example, Schlochman, M.: *Ann. Int. Med.*, 46:728, 1957). Power is strictly a relative term and does not always connote complete success.

Now, every food factor, certainly every vitamin, prevents what it relieves. Thus, we use vitamin C to prevent scurvy because it cures scurvy, and vitamin D to prevent rickets because it cures rickets, and vitamin K to prevent haemorrhagic disease of the newborn because it cures it, and vitamin A to prevent xerophthalmia because it cures it, and vitamin B_1 to prevent neuritis because it cures it, and nicotinic acid to prevent pellagra because it cures it, and riboflavin to prevent glossitis and cheilosis because it cures them, and so on. Thus one uses other food factors such as iron or calcium. Could vitamin E be the sole exception to such a rule?

Admittedly, congenital anomalies are produced long before their recognition and therefore before the average person thinks of treatment, much less of prevention. But there is a great deal of experimental evidence now to indicate that such defects may be the end-result of vitamin deficiencies or hypoxia in the mother at an early stage of embryonic life; we ourselves have published work in this field. See:

J. Ob. & Gyn. Br. Emp., **64**:390, 1957.
Fertility and Sterility, **9**:256, 1958.

It has been concluded that oxygen deficiency in early pregnancy is *the* single most important causative factor in producing anomalies. Obviously, this makes a place for the most powerful physiological oxygenating factor, vitamin E. See:

Tedeschi, C. G., and Ingalls, T. H. (U.S.A.): *Am. J. Ob. & Gyn.*, **71**:16, 1956.

and later Ingalls papers. It may well be that congenital heart disease will prove preventable by means of such nutritional factors as vitamin E. No one must rule out such a possibility prematurely, since it is so likely.

Inflammatory heart lesions like those seen in rheumatic fever follow assaults by a particular strain of streptococcus—but not always, perhaps not commonly. Why? Because of certain unknown factors in resistance. Why do some rheumatic infections recur and many do not? Because of some unknown factors in resistance. Our own experience with the influence of vitamin E on early, primary cases of acute rheumatic fever has occasionally been so dramatic that we ascribe to it considerable powers of increasing such resistance. Moreover, the Aschoff-like nodules seen in the myocardium of vitamin E-deficient calves dying of heart failure would strongly reinforce this view. Holman produced an acute necrotizing arteritis in dogs in relation to kidney damage and vitamin E deficiency. The *J.A.M.A.* commented on this editorially by saying that acute necrotizing arteritis in dogs has a close human counterpart in periarteritis nodosa and rheumatic arteritis in man (*J.A.M.A.*, **137**:1228, 1948). It can be rheumatic lesion, for otherwise the cause of rheumatic fever remains an enigma (*J.A.M.A.*, **171**:1205, 1959).

Atherosclerotic lesions such as those so regularly seen in

:oronary disease and hypertensive states are theoretically preventable by vasodilators, anti-clotting and fibrinolytic agents, if
we accept Duguid's well-attested theory of the origin of atherosclerosis:

Duguid, J. B., and Robertson, W. B. (England): *Lancet,* 1:525,
    1955.
Levene, C. I. (England): *Ibid.,* 2:1216, 1955.
Astrup, T. (Denmark): *Ibid.,* 2:565, 1956.

Here the ingestion of a lasting vasodilator and anti-clotting
and fibrinolytic agent such as alpha tocopherol should provide
the best available prophylaxis. We believe it does, and the Weitzel
studies bear this out.

The references here support the view that vitamin E is helpful in arteriosclerosis:

Ingelman-Sundberg, A. (Sweden): *Acta Endocrinol.,* 2:335, 1949.
Dowd, G. C. (U.S.A.): *Ann. N.Y. Acad. Sci.,* 52:365, 1949.
Merlen, J. F. (France): *Therapie,* 4:262, 1949.
Sterzi, G. (Italy): *Archiv. Ital di Dermat., Sifil. e Venereol.,* 23:257,
    1950.
Galeone, A., and Boero, F. (Italy): *Acta Gerontol.,* 1:3, 1951.
Osten, W. (Germany): *Sonder, aus Internat. Zeits. f. Vitamin-
    forsch.,* 26:19, 1955.
Cali, A., and Adinolfi, M. (Italy): *Gior. Gerontol.,* 3:464, 1955.
Weitzel, G., Schon, H., and Gey, F. (Germany): *Klin. Woch.,*
    33:772, 1955.
Weitzel, G., Schon, H., Gey, F., and Buddecke, E. (Germany):
    Z. Physiol. Chem., Hoppe-Seyler's, 304:247, 1956.
Aslan, A. (Roumania): *Med. Klin.,* 52:1758, 1957.
Szirmai, E. (Hungary): Personal Communication.
Kern, W., Meissner, O., and Spies, R. (Austria): *Wien. med. Woch.,*
    108:175, 1958.
Guillemin, P. (France): *Rev. du Practicien,* 8:1662, 1958.

Moreover, at the moment, American medical men generally
are giving their arteriosclerotic patients more unsaturated fats
(vegetable fats) in their diets as prophylaxis against further
arteriosclerosis. Sternberg has shown that all such diets high in
unsaturated fats require vitamin E as well in order to stabilize

and utilize them properly. Vitamin E preserves them in the bowel:

Sternberg, J., and Pascoe-Dawson, E. (Canada): *Can. M.A.J.* 80:266, 1959.

There appears to be no practical hope for the prevention of cardiovascular disease unless the mechanisms we have sketched above are fundamentally sound and point in the direction of truth. They must not be laughed out of court prematurely, in the way that Jenner's vaccination against smallpox, or Pasteur's vaccination against rabies, or Sabin's oral vaccine against polio has been.

Practically every cardiac and vascular disease state is associated with obstructed blood vessels or a lack of oxygen. Even patients with congestive failure show stasis in the bloodstream and hypoxia. It is self-evident that a key to the treatment of these conditions is the effort to relieve these difficulties, and, apart from the odd surgical procedure such as thrombarterectomy there is no rival to vitamin E in these respects. None can be suggested, indeed, for its oxygen-conserving powers are unique amongst physiological substances, and it acts upon many types of vascular obstruction that the rival anticoagulants do little or nothing to benefit—for example, Buerger's disease, claudication, established thrombus. The references are seen elsewhere in this text.

IS ALPHA TOCOPHEROL AN ANTICOAGULANT?

Several workers have suggested that vitamin E is a natural antithrombin in the bloodstream. The references (cited above also) are:

Zierler, K. L., Grob, D., and Lilienthal, J. L. (U.S.A.): *Am. J Physiol.*, 153:127, 1948.
Kay, J. H., Hutton, S. B., Weiss, G. H., and Ochsner, A. (U.S.A.) *Surgery*, 28:124, 1950.

Whether the observations of such able workers are accurate or not, this is one theory designed to explain the action of vita min E in preventing blood clotting in the bloodstream, something that has always been puzzling. The action on blood clotting of the classical anticoagulants is often puzzling, too, of course, for many patients clot with normal prothrombin times, and there may even be myocardial infarcts without any evidence of an apical thrombus (Branwood, A. W., and Montgomery, G. L.: *Scottish M.J.*, 1:367, 1956). Alpha tocopherol is not the only anti-clotting agent incompletely understood.

It is generally realized by every medical man that its rival anticoagulants, such as heparin or dicumarol, are dangerous. Hence the need to do at least weekly prothrombin tests on every patient taking anticoagulants. Hence the cases of haemorrhage after their use seen every day in every city in the land. Hence the cautious approach of such medical experts as Littman:

Littman, D. (U.S.A.): *New Eng. J. of Med.*, 247:205, 1952.

One would have expected the usual anticoagulants to have been replaced long ago by alpha tocopherol, which is so much safer, and even more effective (since it attacks existing clots as well as prevents further clotting, and minimizes embolism).

ALPHA TOCOPHEROL IN WOUNDS AND BURNS

Vitamin E accelerates the healing of wounds and burns. Since the vascular aspects of these problems are so fundamental, we have included them here—as examples of the stimulation of *normal* circulation by alpha tocopherol. This observation of ours has been confirmed by:

Bartolomucci, E. (Italy): *Archiv. Ital. di Chirurg.*, 50:243, 1938.
Boschi, E., and Gaspari, A. (Italy): *Acta Chir. Potavi*, 7:387, 1951.
Weidenbach, W. (Germany): *Therap. Gegenwart.*, 9:347, 1952.
Block, M. T. (U.S.A.): *Clin. Med.*, 60:1, 1953.
Kohlschmidt, J. (Germany): *Monats. Veterinar.*, 9:157, 1954.
Gualdi, G. (Italy): *Boll. Soc. Med. Clin.*, 54:460, 1954.
Musini (Italy): *Proc. 3rd Internat. Cong. Vit. E,* Venice, Italy, 1955.

We have many photographs of burned and wounded patients to verify such reports.

This observation of ours could be of enormous significance to the population of the United States under atomic attack, when hospitals and medical and nursing personnel are apt to be destroyed or at least overworked. The danger from burns is now our paramount danger, if Hiroshima be any criterion. Some simple, cheap, safe, and self-applicable treatment is needed for survival. Vitamin E is the only one yet suggested.

For our part, we wrote to the Secretary of Defense of the United States and his opposite numbers in England and Canada some years since to bring this most significant observation to their attention. We felt this to be our patriotic duty. Alpha tocopherol might still contain the terrifying men about to leap from the wooden horse. Why let them sweep through our cities unresisted?

ALPHA TOCOPHEROL IN INDOLENT ULCERS

Chronic leg ulcers, whether stasis ulcers or ischaemic ulcers, respond well to alpha tocopherol therapy, particularly if tocopherol ointment is applied locally at the same time. Hot compresses may be used to clean up the sloughing surface, and elevation may occasionally be required. But handled thus, few come to grafting, and those which do need it get better takes. There are many supportive papers in the literature:

Leranth, G., and Frank, L. (Hungary): *Orv. Hetil.,* 80:778, 1938.

Lindgren, I. (Sweden): *Nord. Med.,* 28:2127, 1945.

Castagna, R., and Impallomeni, G. (Italy): *Bol. Soc. Piemont Chir.,* 18:155 (Mar.-May, 1948).

Burgess, J. F., and Pritchard, J. E. (Canada): *Can. M.A.J.,* 59:242, 1948.

Dowd, G. C. (U.S.A.): *Ann. N.Y. Acad. of Sci.,* 52:365, 1949.

Siedentopf, H., and Kruger, A. (Germany): *Sonder. med. Klin.,* 44:1060, 1949.

Guerrini, G., and Bonanome, A. (Italy): *Arch. Att. Soc. Ital. Chir.,* 51st Congress, 1949.

Garetta (France): Thesis, Toulouse #91, 1949.

Comi, G., and Nesi, G. (Italy): *Riv. Crit. di Clin. Med.,* 50:214, 1950.

Block, M. T. (U.S.A.): *Clin. Med.*, 57:112, 1950.

de Graciansky, P., and Boule, S. (France): *Bull. de la Soc. Franc. de Dermatol. et de Syphil.*, 2:213, 1950.

Owings, J. C. (U.S.A.): See discussions—Ochsner, A., Kay, J. H., De Camp, P. T., Hutton, S. B., and Balla, G. A.: *Ann. Surg.*, 131:652, 1950.

Hagerman, G. (Sweden): *Archiv. f. Dermat. u. Syphil.*, 191:637, 1950.

Bierzynski, A. (West Indies): *Caribbean M.J.*, 12:5, 1950.

Sterzi, F. (Italy): *Archiv. Ital. di Dermat., Sifil. e Venereol.*, 23:257, 1950.

Bijdendijk, A., and Noordhoek, F. J. (Holland): *Neder Tijd. v. Geneeskunde,* 95:1039, 1951.

Coatsworth, R. C. (Canada): *Summary,* 3:1, 1951.

Garcia, G. C. (Spain): *Med. Española,* 25:345, 1951.

Wegner, A. (Germany): *Dermatol. Woch.*, 123:385, 1951.

Walther, H. (Germany): *Hautarzt,* 2:526, 1951.

Schmid, S. (Austria): *Wien. klin. Woch.*, 64:128, 1952.

Lohel, H. (Germany): *Deutsche Gesund.*, 7:1365, 1952.

Grubb, E. (Sweden): *Acta Dermatol. Venereol.*, 32:256, 1952.

Bonaccorsi, R., and Vicari, F. (Italy): *Riv. di Patol. e Clin.*, 7:469, 1952.

Block, M. T. (U.S.A.): *Clin. Med.*, 60:1, 1953.

Lee, M. (England): *Brit. J. Dermatol.*, 65:131, 1953.

Gaumond, E. (Canada): *L'Union Med. du Canada,* 82:141, 1953.

Della Thommasa, F. (Italy): *Gazz. med. Ital.*, 113:256, 1954.

Kohlschmidt, J. (Germany): *Monats. Veterinarmed.*, 9:157, 1954.

Sacino, G. (Italy): *Minerva Med.*, 45:1145, 1954.

Osten, W. (Germany): *Sonder aus. Internat. Zeits. f. Vitaminforsch.*, 26:19, 1955.

de Angelis (Italy): *Arch. dermatol. exp. e functionale,* 5:53, 1955.

de Angelis, G. (Italy)—quoted by M. Comel (Italy): *Proc. 3rd Internat. Cong. on Vit. E,* Venice, Sept., 1955, p. 404.

Lee, M. (England): *Ibid.,* p. 445.

Salomon, A. (Holland): *Separat. aus du Ars Medici,* 8:1547, 1956.

Nikolowski, W. (Germany): *Parfumerie u. Kosmetic,* 8:1, 1956.

Sturm, W. (Germany): Reported at Congress for Spa- and Physical Therapy, Bad Elster, Germany, Oct. 25, 1956.

Guillemin, P. (France): *Rev. du Praticien,* 8:1662, 1958.

Barabasch, M. E. (U.S.S.R.): *Vestnik Dermatol i. Venereol.*, 32:31, 1958.

Frey, I. G. (Germany): *Strahlentherapie,* 95:440, 1959.

ALPHA TOCOPHEROL IN COLLAGENOSIS

Chronic brawny induration of the lower leg, usually on the basis of old phlebitis and chronic venous stasis, often associated with stubborn ulceration, is not remedied by the use of alpha tocopherol. Nothing can undo the scarring these legs display. But the process, which usually extends so inexorably till it girdles first one leg and then the other, comes to a full stop on adequate alpha tocopherol therapy. If it extends it merely means that not enough tocopherol is being administered. Here at last is an effective answer to a debilitating and painful vascular problem for which nothing has ever been suggested before but the most drastic, tedious and ugly surgery.

The so-called varicose eczema so often associated with it often responds well to the local application of tocopherol ointment. One must be cautious and slow in applying it, lest it spread the rash elsewhere.

ALPHA TOCOPHEROL IN VARICOSE VEINS

We never advise surgery for varicose veins unless for cosmetic reasons in women. Otherwise alpha tocopherol can give as good a final result as operation, since the latter is so regularly followed by recurrence in about 1½ years' time. Alpha tocopherol increases collateral circulation around the deep, obstructed veins, decreases ankle oedema and leg ache, halts the varicose process, cuts down or relieves any associated skin irritation, and lets the patient walk much better. Often the veins seem to regress, although this is unpredictable.

ALPHA TOCOPHEROL AS A VASODILATOR

Vitamin E is universally believed to be a vasodilator. We first demonstrated this years ago, but the observation has been supported by casual reference in nearly every paper on the vascular uses of vitamin E, and specifically by the following investigators:

Rietti, M. F. (Italy): *Presse Med.*, **56**:870, 1948.
Tusini, G. (Italy): *Boll. Soc. Lomb. Sci. Med. Biol.*, March 15, 1949.

Seidenari, R., Mars, G., and Morpurgo, M. (Italy): *Acta Gerontol.,* 1:55, 1951.

Enria, G., and Fererro, R. (Italy): *Arch. per la Sci. Med.,* 91:23, 1951.

Edgerton, M. T., Hanrahan, E. M., and Davis, W. B. (U.S.A.): *Plastic & Reconstruc. Surg.,* 8:224, 1951.

Walther, H. (Germany): *Hautarzt,* 2:526, 1951.

Sabatini, C., and Tagliavini, R. (Italy): *Proc. 2nd Nat. Cong. on Gerontol. & Geriat.,* Milan, March, 1952.

ten Berge, B. S., and Polak, R. (Holland): *First World Cong. on Fertility and Sterility,* New York, May, 1953.

d'Ardes, V. (Italy): *Gazz. med. Ital.,* 112:190, 1953.

Schmitt, A., and Luzius, H. (Germany): *Aertsliche Forsch.,* 8:45, 1954.

Zampetti, C. A. (Italy): *Proc. 3rd Internat. Cong. on Vit. E,* Venice, 1955.

Bottiglioni, E., and Sturani, P. L. (Italy): *Ibid.*

Kern, H., Meissner, O., and Spies, R. (Austria): *Wien. med. Woch.,* 108:175, 1958.

One of the earliest and most dramatic experiments in this group is that of Tusini, who produced vasospasm in the tail artery of a rat by means of ergotamine tartrate, then released the same with vitamin E.

On any other grounds it is difficult to explain the good results obtained in the tocopherol treatment of intermittent claudication:

Keleman, E., and Lajos, I. (Hungary): *Orvosok Lapja,* 4:1603, 1948.

Leinwand, I. (U.S.A.): *N.Y. State J. Med.,* 48:1503, 1948.

Guerrini, G., and Bonanome, A. (Italy): *Arch. Att. Soc. Ital. Chir.,* 51st Cong., 1949.

de Oliviera, D. (Brazil): *Separata de O Hopital,* July, 1949.

Boyd, A. M., Ratcliffe, A. H., Jepson, R. P., and James, G. W. H. (England): *(Br.) J. Bone & Joint Surg.,* 31:325, 1949.

Comi, G., and Nesi, C. (Italy): *Riv. Crit. de Clin. Med.,* 50:214, 1950.

Butturini, U. (Italy): *Gior. de Clin. Med.,* 31:1, 1950.

Galeone, A., and Minelli, M. (Italy): *Minerva Med.,* 46:694, 1950.

Boyd, A. M. (England): *Brit. Med. J.,* 2:112, 1951.

Heinsen, H. A., and Scheffler, H. (Germany): *Med. Woch.,* 46:909, 1951.

Schmid, S. (Austria): *Wien. klin. Woch.,* 64:128, 1952.

Dalla Torre, L., and Boldrini, R. (Italy): *Clin. Nuova,* 12:617, 1952.

Bonaccorsi, R., and Vicari, F. (Italy): *Riv. di patol. e Clin.,* 7:469, 1952.

Boyd, A. M., Hall Ratcliffe, A., and Bloor, K. (England): *Lancet,* 1:491, 1953.

d'Ardes, V. (Italy): *Gazz. med. Ital.,* 112:190, 1953.

Osten, W. (Germany): *Sonder. aus Internat. zeits. f. Vitamin,* 26:19, 1955.

Bottiglioni, E., and Sturani, P. L. (Italy): *Proc. 3rd Internat. Cong. Vit. E,* Venice, 1955.

Livingstone, P. D., and Jones, C. (England): *Lancet,* 2:602, 1958.

Guillemin, P. (France): *Rev. du Practicien,* 8:1662, 1958.

Even more graphic are the beautiful demonstrations by Enria and Fererro and the Dominguez team:

Enria, G., and Fererro, R. (Italy): *Arch. per la Sci. Med.,* 91:23, 1951.

Dominguez, J. P., and Dominguez, R. (Spain): *Angiologia,* 5:51, 1953.

The first of these tied off the femoral vein in dogs and then administered alpha tocopherol, obtaining great vasodilatation of collateral vessels. The Dominguez team did the same thing after tieing off the femoral artery in rabbits; they reported that some of the collaterals dilated to larger size than the original femoral artery!

May we add that alpha tocopherol is remarkably helpful in Raynaud's syndrome on just this same basis, as it is in varicose eczema, Buerger's disease, and such conditions.

ALPHA TOCOPHEROL AND ROENTGEN TISSUE INJURY

Vitamin E has been used to treat x-ray burns. We discussed such results at the Second World Congress on Vitamin E at New York in 1949 (see *Ann. N.Y. Acad. Sci.,* 52:358, 1949).

Since that time there has been abundant confirmation:

Herve, A., and Bacq, Z. M. (France): *Compt. Rend. Soc. Biol.,* 143:1158, 1949.

Block, M. T. (U.S.A.): *Clin. Med.*, 57:112, 1950.
Pascher, F., Sawicky, H. H., Silverberg, H. G., Braitman, M., and
    Karoff, N. B. (U.S.A.): *J. Investigative Derm.*, 17:261, 1951.
Bacq, Z. M. (France): *Experientia*, 7:11, 1951.
Kemmer, C. H. (Germany): *Dermatol. Woch.*, 125:1209, 1952.
Lohel, H. (Germany): *Deutsche Gesund.*, 7:1365, 1952.
Sabatini, C., Balli, L., and Tagliavini, R. (Italy): *Radiol. Med.*,
    39:1201, 1953.
Hutter (Germany): *Deutsche Gesund.*, 9:277, 1954.
Frey, I. G. (Germany): *Strahlentherapie*, 95:440, 1954.
Barabasch, M. E. (U.S.S.R.): *Vestnik. Dermatol. i. Venereol.*,
    32:31, 1958.

As has been stressed above, this use of alpha tocopherol promises to be one of the most important roles it has in the medical management of injuries incurred in atomic warfare. There has been no other suggestion as practical and simple and cheap. Indeed, there has been no other suggestion. We regard this as our most salutary discovery.

ALPHA TOCOPHEROL AND DIABETES MELLITUS

It has never been suggested that vitamin E was a "cure" for diabetes, any more than Banting claimed insulin as a "cure." It is indispensable treatment, however.

Long years after the discovery of insulin, it is recognized that it and dietary restriction control high blood sugar levels—but that many or all long-treated diabetics go on to display degeneration of the eyes, kidneys, heart, and peripheral vessels. Hence the common finding of cataracts, retinitis, Kimmelstiel-Wilson kidney, coronary attacks, and leg gangrene in long-treated diabetics. The greatest American authority, Joslin, has twice commented on this—see *J.A.M.A.*, 147:209, 1951. More recently (*J.A.M.A.*, 156:1584, 1954) he said that insulin hid the tragic symptoms and signs of diabetes and thus allowed slowly developing arteriosclerosis to kill the patient. Doctors cannot afford to have 85 per cent of their patients begin to have disease of the kidney, heart, and brain and begin to grow blind after the disease has lasted only 15 years. Only one in 10 patients is now eligible for a life expectancy medal for living longer with diabetes than expected to live without it, and only 54 in the world have been found perfect after 25 years of the disease. Surely doctors should be able to postpone the onset of complications until after 15 years in more than 15 per cent of their cases.

Obviously, therefore, diet and insulin leave much to be desired still. An increasing number of diabetic specialists now recognize that diabetes is a two-phase disease, one being related to hyperglycaemia and the other to vascular degeneration (Downie, E., and Martin, F. R. (Australia): *Diabetes,* 8:383, 1959). All that insulin treatment has done is to clear away the high blood sugar to reveal the second phase.

Vitamin E has long been known to heal some of the vascular complications of diabetes and even decrease the need for insulin. The references are numerous:

Butturini, U. (Italy): *Gior. di Clin. Med.,* **26**:90, 1945.

Molotchick, M. B. (U.S.A.): *Med. Rec.,* **160**:667, 1947.

Doumer, E., Merlen, J., and Dubruille, P. (France): *Presse Med.,* 29:394, 1949.

Merlen, J. F. (France): *Therapie,* 4:262, 1949.

Guerrini, G., and Bonanome, A. (Italy): *Arch. Atti. Soc. Ital. Chir.,* 51st Cong., 1949.

Butturini, U. (Italy): *Gior. di Clin. Med.,* 31:1, 1950.

Dietrich, H. W. (U.S.A.): *South. M.J.,* 43:743, 1950.

Block, M. T. (U.S.A.): *Clin. Med.,* 57:112, 1950.

Butturini, U., and Baronchelli, A. (Italy): *Boll. Soc. Ital. Biol. Sper.,* 26:744, 1950.

Charalampous, F. C., and Hegsted, D. M. (U.S.A.): *Am. J. Physiol.,* 161:540, 1950.

Levene, H. E., and Rosgen, M. (Germany): *Munch. med. Woch.,* 92:339, 1950.

Ged (France): *Med. Thesis,* Sim, Paris, 1951, #471.

Edgerton, M. T., Hanrahan, E. M., and Davis, W. B. (U.S.A.): *Plastic & Reconstructive Surg.,* 8:224, 1951.

George, N. (Canada): *Summary,* 3:74, 1951.

Terzani, C. (Italy): *Policlinica—Sezione Prat.,* 58:1381, 1951.

Coatsworth, R. C. (Canada): *Summary,* 3:25, 1951.

Yener, M. S. (Turkey): *Turk. Tip. Cemiyeti Mecmuasi,* **17**:70, 1951.

Day, R. (U.S.A.): *Southern M.J.*, 44:549, 1951.

Mosetti, A., and Boesi, S. (Italy): *Med. Internazionale*, 60:210, 1952.

Feraboli, P. C. (Italy): *Gazz. med. Ital.*, 111:285, 1952.

Pareja, C. A. (Ecuador): *Gaz. Med. Ecuador*, 7:3, 1952.

Massobrio, E., and Boglione, G. (Italy): *Arch. per le Sci. Med.*, 77:263, 1952.

Block, M. T. (U.S.A.): *Clin. Med.*, 60:1, 1953.

d'Ardes, V. (Italy): *Gazz. med. Ital.*, 112:190, 1953.

Gounelle, H., Marnay, C., and Rabii, H. (France): *Presse Med.*, 62:888, 1954.

Romeo, F., and Parrinello, A. (Italy): *Acta Vitaminol.*, 8:129, 1954.

Benacchio, L. (Italy): *Il policlinico*, 62:486, 1955.

Bottiglioni, E., and Sturani, P. L. (Italy): *Proc. 3rd Internat. Cong. Vit. E*, Venice, 1955.

Rodriguez, C. F. A. (Peru): *Am. Fac. Farm. Bioquim., Lima*, 7:421, 1956.

Sturm, W. (Germany): Read before Congress on Spa- and Physical Therapy, Bad Elster, Germany, October 25, 1956.

Lee, Pei-fei (U.S.A.): *Summary*, 8:85, 1957.

Gargello, E. C., and Merlo, M. A. (Spain): *Rev. Clin. Española*, 69:25, 1958.

Guillemin, P. (France): *Rev. du Practicien*, 8:1662, 1958.

We published photographs of diabetic and other gangrenes treated with vitamin E in an issue of the *Canadian Medical Association Journal* a few years ago:

Tolgyes, S., and Shute, E. V. (Canada): *Can. M.A.J.*, 76:730, 1957.

No one can deny that vitamin E is an important and useful therapeutic agent in the management of diabetes. Indeed, several of the papers above suggest that it lowers blood sugars as well as improves the vascular half of the disease. For example, Tolgyes found that this occurred in about 25 per cent of cases he treated.

Tolgyes, S. (Canada): *Summary*, 9:7, 1957.

ALPHA TOCOPHEROL IN FOOD SHOULD BE DISCUSSED, FINALLY

If any food, including vitamin E, ceases to be taken, any effect it has produced on the body soon wears off. This is true of potatoes or iron or calcium or fat or carbohydrates or proteins or vitamin B or vitamin D. Some of these items are held or stored by the body longer than others, but all nutrients are soon utilized by the body and burned up or excreted and need to be replaced unless any nutritional effects so produced are to be minimized. This is our reason for eating regularly, perhaps three times daily. It is a truism, indeed.

The maximum tocopherol level in the blood attained after the ingestion of vitamin E is reached in 4 to 8 hours, after which serum levels tail off to their pre-existing levels in about 72 hours. The evidence for this comes from such studies as:

Beckman, R. (Germany): *Zeits. f. Vitamin-Hormone & Enzyme Studies,* 7:153, 1955.
Rindi, G., and Perri, V. (Italy): *Internat. Rev. of Vit. Res.,* 28:274, 1958.
Sternberg, J., and Pascoe-Dawson, E. (Canada): *Can. M.A.J.,* 80:266, 1959.

Thus, Beckmann has shown that if one takes 100 mgm. of alpha tocopherol the blood values revert to normal in 24 hours. If 400 mgm. are given the blood level of tocopherol in 24 hours is only 22 per cent higher than its previous values.

Long ago we came to the same conclusion on purely clinical grounds, and published our views.

For a long time now, some authorities have been saying that "the need for tocopherols in human nutrition has not been established." Suddenly they have been ejected from this palpably false position by studies reported on October 30 in Washington newspapers (and dating from an order signed on October 23, 1959, by F.D.A. Commissioner Larrick). We are pleased to see the American Food and Drug Administration compelled to reverse its long stand in this matter by American workers like Horwitt—and *after* the uselessness of vitamin E in human nutrition had been emphasized officially for two decades.

Another old chestnut is that the average Canadian or American diet is adequate in vitamin E and needs no supplementation. The corollary of this is that "the North American is not vitamin

E-deficient. He has lived on normal intakes and still does." Nothing could be farther from the facts.

It may be possible that the mythical North American has an adequate intake of mixed tocopherols or, in medical slang, "vitamin E." But only one of these, the *alpha* tocopherol, appears to have major nutritional and medical significance. It is quite disingenuous for nutritional "authorities" to quote the total tocopherol content of foods in an effort to show that they contain enough *alpha* tocopherol. Only the alpha tocopherol content can ever be a medical issue. Only alpha tocopherol is the League of Nations standard. *To almost all investigators in the field alpha tocopherol is the only subject of discussion.*

Studies on bottle-fed infants indicate that they require 2.5 to 5.0 mgm. d-alpha-tocopherol daily. They get 0.3 to 0.7 mgm. daily in a 24 oz. feeding, however. Horwitt more recently has concluded that 30 mgm. per day is needed by an adult living on the average American high fat diet. Engel and Harris had earlier come to that identical conclusion. They further calculated the average Dutch or American intake at 14 to 15 mgm. daily. Harris points out that even this value is too high because based on vitamin determinations in fresh, raw foods, not yet processed, stored or cooked; it pays no attention to the degree of assimilation by different persons. Hickman has calculated that the average American adult requires 20 to 170 mgm. of alpha tocopherol daily (Fall Issue of *Record of Chemical Progress,* 1948). He estimated that his actual intake is about 6 to 13 mgm. daily. Indeed, the diets suggested by the United States National Research Council contain 6 mgm. of alpha tocopherol per day, and much of this is destroyed in cooking, by association with unsaturated fats in other foods ingested at the same time, or by inorganic iron, and so on. Deep-frying, for example, destroys 70 to 90 per cent of alpha tocopherol and baking pies 25 to 75 per cent (see Quaife, M. L. (U.S.A.): *J. Nutrit.,* **40:**367, 1950). It may be that the average American really absorbs each day only 3 to 5 mgm. of alpha tocopherol—much less than any estimate of his daily requirement.

Mackenzie, J. B. (U.S.A.): *Pediatrics,* 13:346, 1954.

Gordon, H. H., Nitowski, H. M., and Cornblatt, M. (U.S.A.): *J. Dis. Child.,* 90:669, 1955.

Gordon, H. H., Nitowski, H. M., Levin, S., and Tilden, J. (U.S.A.): *Internat. Cong. Pediat.,* July 19–25, 1959, p. 118.

Horwitt, M. K. (U.S.A.): *Am. J. Clin. Nutrit.* (in press).

Engel, C. (Holland): *Ann. N.Y. Acad. Sci.,* 52:292, 1949.

Harris, P. L. (U.S.A.): *Ibid.,* 52:240, 1949.

Wright, S. W., Filer, L. J., and Mason, K. E. (U.S.A.): *Pediatrics,* 7:386, 1951.

Harris, P. L., Quaife, M. L., and Swanson, W. J. (U.S.A.): *J. Nutrit.,* 40:164, 1950.

Now every animal but the goat which has been given alpha tocopherol-deficient diets sooner or later develops heart damage, usually a focal necrosis of the muscle wall, often associated with electrocardiographic changes indicating myocardial damage, and sometimes, as in calves or cows, ending in sudden cardiac failure and death. Is it possible that the human heart muscle is so different that it can withstand decades of *almost complete alpha* tocopherol withdrawal and survive these decades unscathed? Almost certainly not.

However, *we want it clearly understood that we have not and do not suggest alpha tocopherol only as replacement therapy,* the sole role originally suggested for vitamins. The idea of using vitamins as biochemical agents per se is now well established and doses of vitamin C or D or of certain vitamin K analogues are regularly used these days in doses *enormously* in excess of "replacement" dosage and for purposes often resembling their supplementary role only distantly. It is *strictly logical and inside current medical tradition,* therefore, to administer alpha tocopherol as *a biochemical agent per se, the dosage levels of such usage having no relationship whatever to the dosage required to substitute for a vitamin deficiency.* It is irrelevant and disingenuous to say that alpha tocopherol has no therapeutic role because no tocopherol deficiency syndrome has been demonstrated in man. (Current experiment seems to be remedying this hiatus in knowledge very rapidly.) Be it remembered that from the first we have spoken of a dosage level in cardiovascular disease of 10 to 100 times the estimated daily requirement. We use alpha tocopherol not as a "vitamin" but as a drug.

There can be *no reasonable doubt* that chronic deficiency of alpha tocopherol (not of "vitamin E") leads to myocardial damage in man. Alpha tocopherol could be used to restore such a deficiency and this probably would help such a damaged cardiovascular system. But *we have steadily used alpha tocopherol as a pharmacodynamic agent in its own right,* and are therefore *quite uninterested in an argument that it should be used only as replacement therapy in small doses, and that in those small doses it is not pharmacologically effective.* This line of thought has long been irrelevant to alpha tocopherol therapy.

INTEREST BEYOND THE IRON CURTAIN

One of the encouraging aspects of tocopherol studies is the current interest of scientists beyond the Iron Curtain who have published a good deal in the field. Some recent papers dealing with the use of vitamin E in cardiovascular disease from beyond the Iron Curtain are:

Kemmer, C. H. (Poland): *Derm. Woch.,* **126**:1209, 1952.
Bruchnerova, O. (Czechoslovakia): *Lokarski listy,* **7**:549, 1952.
Vitak, B. (Czechoslovakia): *Cesko, Gynaek.,* **19**:345, 1954.
Bruchnerova, O. (Czechoslovakia): *Vintrni lekarstvi,* **1**:137, 1955.
Kliment, Deak, and Kovalchikova (Czechoslovakia): *Cesko, Gynaek.,* **22**:67, 1957.
Aslan, A. (Roumania): *Med. Klin.,* **52**:1758, 1957.
Barwick-Schramm, A., and Mol, A. (Poland): *Polski Arch. Med. Wewnet.,* **27**:301, 1957.
Szirmai, E. (Hungary): *Summary,* **10**:87, 1958.
Szirmai, E. (Hungary): *Zeits. f. ges. innr. Med.,* **13**:479, 1958.
Anisimov, V. E. (U.S.S.R.): *Klinich. Meditsina,* **36**:147, 1958.
Barabasch, M. E. (U.S.S.R.): *Vestnik. Dermatol. i. Venereol.,* **32**:31, 1958.

—in addition to many other reports on the use of vitamin E in allied fields of medicine. Indeed, Russian workers have suggested that it be added to food in restaurants. (Berezovskaya, N. N., et al.: *Voprosy Pitaniya,* 15:37, 1956).

SUMMARY

A general review is presented, indicating some of the reasoning now standing behind the use of alpha tocopherol in cardiovascular disease, and stressing particularly its use as a pharmacodynamic agent, not merely its administration as "replacement" or "vitamin" therapy.

Appendix B

The Vitamin E Controversy

Reprinted from "How to Eat for a Healthy Heart," by J. I. Rodale, Rodale Books, and published in Prevention *Magazine, March, 1963.*

In the *American Journal of Physiology,* 153:127, 1948, K. L. Zierler, D. Grob, and J. L. Lilienthal describe experiments in which they discovered that vitamin E has a profound effect on the blood, especially its clotting qualities. It has a strong anticlotting effect both in laboratory experiments and in the veins and arteries of human beings. Now there is a special natural substance in the blood called heparin which is made in the liver, whose job it is to prevent the coagulation of blood. In their tests these scientists found that the action of vitamin E on the blood takes place regardless of how much or how little heparin is present in the blood stream of the patients. So there can be no doubt that the anticoagulating action is the result of the vitamin E and nothing else.

In the case of a thrombosis, or heart attack by means of a blood clot, the taking of sufficient vitamin E can save lives, by preventing the blood from forming clots. A standard practice in certain heart cases is to administer the drug heparin for this purpose, but vitamin E has other purposes also and is a much more valuable and safer tool.

In the Italian journal, *Bollettino Societa Chirurgia,* 18:155 (1948), R. Castagna and G. Impallomeni report on 7 patients with phlebitis (inflammation of a vein) and one 71-year-old woman who had had an ulcer measuring 5 by 3 inches on her lower leg. The phlebitis responded dramatically to the use of vitamin E alone. The woman patient's ulcer healed in 20 days. The authors have also used vitamin E in treatment of vascular disease (any disease of the blood vessels) and for "strokes." They tell us that in thrombophlebitis (inflammation of the vein in which a blood clot is involved) the improvement by using vitamin E is extremely rapid. In addition, they say, treatment with vitamin E does not require a rigid blood control as do other medications.

From Brazil (*Publication of the O Hospital* for July, 1949) D. de Olivera describes 2 cases of phlebitis, one during a pregnancy and one following childbirth. In both cases, fever fell rapidly and there was no occurrence of the disease when the first patient had her child. The British medical publication, *The Lancet,* 2:132, 1949, carries an article by A. M. Boyd, A. H. James, and G. W. H. and R. P. Jepson, saying that clinical results with vitamin E are far better than any obtained with any other treatment in cases of obliterative diseases of the blood vessels. It can be used most successfully for the relief of cramps in the calves of the legs. "May we repeat," say these authors, "that it is our considered opinion that the clinical observations so far made warrant the continued use of vitamin E therapy."

A Norwegian physician, H. Sturup, writing in *Nordisk Medicin,* 43:721, 1950, tells us he has seen a number of cases of thrombosis helped by vitamin E therapy. He discusses in detail the case of a 33-year-old patient who had chronic phlebitis of the left leg, 5 years after an operation. This patient was not even confined to bed, but took vitamin E daily and within 6 days the pain and swelling disappeared.

The Annals of Surgery, 131:652, reports that vitamin E and calcium appear to be helpful in the treatment of vascular diseases. Dr. A. W. Allen of Boston, commenting on this article, tells us that he had used vitamin E on a number of patients and can report that 50 of these who were "vulnerable," that is susceptible, to thrombosis, escaped this serious condition. This seems to us particularly important, for in these cases vitamin E was used to prevent rather than to cure, and 50 lucky patients continued in good health. Dr. J. C. Owings, of Baltimore, comments that he has treated many leg ulcers due to phlebitis with a combination of rutin and vitamin E, all of which remained healed, so long as the patient continued to take the vitamin.

Postgraduate Medicine, 10:794, 1951, carries a report by A. Ochsner who believes that vitamin E is the best preventive of a blood clot, because it is a natural substance, and there is no hazard involved in its use. The use of other anticoagulants is dangerous and tying off veins should not be practiced because it will not protect against the detachment of clots. He states that he does not know whether vitamin E combined with calcium is the final answer, but adds that it seems to be best, because it is perfectly safe and does not bring any danger of producing bleeding.

Medical Thesis, published in Paris, No. 471, 1951, quotes a physician as saying he has found vitamin E and calcium useful for preventing blood clots after surgery. R. Bauer, writing in *Wiene Klinisch Wochenschrift,* a German publication, 31:552, 1951, says Dr. Ochsner's method can be used successfully in reducing to one-tenth of the usual incidence of thrombosis and should perhaps be used to decrease the danger of clot in coronary thrombosis. M. Reifferscheid and P. Matis, writing in *Medizinische Welt,* Germany, 20:1168, 1951, announce they have found vitamin E to be definitely protective against vascular clotting. They found that large daily doses were necessary. They describe 5 cases of diabetic gangrene, 9 cases of Raynaud's disease (a gangrenous condition), 7 cases of Dupuytren's contracture (contraction of tissues under the skin of the palm), and 14 cases of hemorrhagic (bleeding) diseases that all yielded to treatment with vitamin E.

Drs. W. E. Crump and E. F. Heiskell, writing in the *Texas State Journal of Medicine,* 11, 1952, agree that the use of the regular anticoagulants for routine prevention of clotting diseases in patients after operations is too dangerous for general use. In most cases where these medicines are used, as many patients die of hemorrhage as might have died of clots and 16 per cent of other cases develop non-fatal bleeding complications. When vitamin E was used as treatment by these physicians, no bleeding occurred and only minor side reactions were noticed. When cases of phlebitis occurred during treatment, they were mild and had no complications. There were no lung clots, fatal or non-fatal, in patients being treated with vitamin E. Dr. Terrel Speed, commenting on these statements, says, "Considerable evidence is accumulating to substantiate the value of this therapy. However, I have gradually expanded its use and now it is used routinely in essentially the same group of cases mentioned by the authors. If the promising preliminary results are borne out, relative protection against one of the most feared complications of surgery will have been obtained."

Two German physicians, S. Schmid writing in *Wiene Klinisch Wochenschrift,* 64, and H. Wagner writing in *Aertzliche Wochenschrift,* 7:248, 1952, say they have achieved good results in treating thrombosis with vitamin E.

In spite of this kind of evidence, accumulated in increasing quantity over the years, some medical journals are still taking pot shots at vitamin E therapy and spreading doubt as to its effectiveness. Such an article appeared in the *British Medical Journal* for December, 1952. It was answered promptly by Drs. Evan S. and Wilfrid E. Shute, the two Canadian doctors who have specialized in the use of vitamin E in the treatment of vascular cases. Say these two doctors: "The leading article on 'The Therapeutic Uses of Vitamin E' (December 20, 1952) certainly calls for comment by us, the proponents of the use of alpha-tocopherol (vitamin E) in cardiovascular disease.

"Such an article might conceivably have been written in 1948 or 1949. However, the picture has changed so rapidly since that time that your leading article now simply does not reflect the findings of investigators in this field. This is best illustrated perhaps by the current issue of our medical journal, *The Summary,* which contains the abstracts of 122 reports which have appeared in the medical literature supporting our original contentions. Since the American Aristotles first condemned it, too many doctors have dropped a pebble from their own towers to make that condemnation stick.

"Briefly, our current *Summary* records that 17 reports have supported us in the use of alpha-tocopherol for the menopause; 5 in its use for nephritis; 6 for kraurosis vulvae; 4 for capillary permeability; 4 for purpura; 5 for vascular dilatation; 11 for Buerger's disease; 10 for vascular sclerosis; 15 for thrombosis; 3 for muscular power; 20 for indolent ulcers; 14 for diabetes; 4 for Roentgen tissue damage; 4 for incipient gangrene; 2 for wound healing. Finally, 46 reports have supported us in the use of alpha-tocopherol for heart disease.

"It is difficult to believe that all these investigators have duplicated an error. Certainly it is cavalier to dismiss such work in one paragraph."

ACTION OF VITAMIN E

I would like to quote from a speech delivered by Dr. Evan Shute of the Shute Foundation of London, Ontario, Canada, to show how vitamin E acts in the body:

"The power of vitamin E to treat and prevent heart disease of all types, whether coronary or rheumatic, depends upon four chief characteristics:

"(1) Vitamin E seems to be a natural anti-thrombin in the human blood stream. It has been found by Zierler of Johns Hopkins and the U.S. Navy Research Department and Kay at Tulane to be a substance normally circulating in the blood of all men which prevents clots occurring inside the vessel. It is the only substance preventing the clotting of blood which is not dangerous. It does not interfere with the normal clotting of blood in a wound and with the normal healing process. Indeed, it actually accelerates the healing of burns and wounds.

"(2) The second important effect of the use of vitamin E is oxygen conservation. It is a natural antioxidant in the body. It has been shown by Houchin and Mattill, and this has been confirmed by many workers, to decrease the oxygen requirement of muscle by as much as 43 per cent and makes the narrow stream of blood which gets through the narrowed coronary artery in many heart patients adequate to prevent the occurrence of anoxia (lack of oxygen), which is the trigger that sets off anginal or heart pain. Consequently, we have patients in Montreal who were once unable to walk half a block without the occurrence of angina pectoris but are now able to climb Mount Royal. Indeed, there is present in my audience today at least one such patient.

"(3) The third major function of vitamin E is the prevention of excessive scar tissue production and even, in some instances, the ability to melt away unwanted scar. It has been proven to function in this way in many areas of the body—from the hand, in Dupuytren's contraction (Rochester, N.Y.)—to urinary tract strictures (Johns Hopkins).

"(4) It is a dilator of blood vessels. This was beautifully demonstrated by x-ray in rabbits injected before and after the administration of vitamin E by two workers in Florence, Italy. It opens up new pathways in the damaged circulation, therefore, and by-passes blocks produced by clots and hardened arteries.

"These four functions, all of them extensively confirmed in animal experimentation and human clinical work, make it the most valuable ally the cardiologist has yet found in the treatment of heart disease. It has no rivals. No other substance has this array of needful properties. This drug then becomes the first safe drug which can be given to patients suffering from the results of a clot in a coronary artery. There has been and still is no treatment at all for this type of case except two mildly useful drugs, which can be administered with great peril to the already precarious patient. Vitamin E replaces 'rest and reassurance,' which have no authentic basis, with real help to the damaged, laboring heart itself. It is the key both to the prevention and treatment of all those conditions in which a lack of blood supply due to thickened or blocked blood vessels or a lack of oxygen is a major part or the whole story of the disease. As I have said, it has no rivals. No pharmacologist or internist can suggest another substance with all the powers and properties of this vitamin. God made it unique and we ignore it at our peril.

"This work is world famous. Some 96 medical papers, not including our own, have already been written in its support. How many does one need to win his case?

"Our work seems to have been the source of Ochsner's studies on the prevention of postoperative clotting by the use of vitamin E, of the work of many Italian workers on heart disease, of Professor Boyd's (of the University of Manchester) published treatment of intermittent claudication (Buerger's disease to you) and with phlebitis; of much recent work on diabetes mellitus. Indeed, the treatment of diabetes mellitus nowadays requires three agents, not two. These are: a balanced diet, insulin, and vitamin E! Any one or two alone are not adequate. The three form a nearly unbeatable combination. Everyone interested in treating diabetes now is aware of the deplorable results achieved by the use of insulin and diet only [except in the U.S.—Ed.].

"We have over 160 medical men as personal patients at our institute. We know of many more who are taking it on their own. Presumably what is good enough for them is good enough for their patients. Early this month one appeared who had been a successful surgeon in California. After a heart attack he had been given vitamin E by his doctor. He merely came to us for regulation of his dosage. He used these words to me. 'Everybody is using it for the treatment of heart disease in California!'—a pleasant but slight exaggeration, perhaps.

"There is much animal experimentation to show that this drug may be the key to the control of hardening of the arteries. I cannot help but recall the words of the great pathologist, Gideon Wells, under whom I studied pathology for 15 months, who told me that the man who discovered the prevention and treatment of arteriosclerosis had found the key to eternal youth. A man is as old or as young as his arteries.

"I would, if I had the time, give you in detail the results of some of these experiments. I could tell you of the work of Tusini in Italy, who showed that a substance like Ergotamine tartrate which caused spasms of the arteries in rats could be neutralized by vitamin E, and that giving vitamin E to the animal ahead of time would protect him against the action of this drug. I would like to tell you about the workers who showed that deposition of cholesterol in the walls of the arteries in rabbits force-fed cholesterol could be prevented by vitamin E.

"We think that vitamin E can safely be added to the list of so-called 'wonder' drugs. No one knows precisely the mode of action of any of these, but that they act and on what they act are matters of common knowledge. It was not always so. It took 14 years from the first investigation of penicillin before it came into general use, but the doctor who was responsible for this is now Lady Florey.

"We are happy to have them instrumental in discovering the use of vitamin E in treating cardiovascular disease, not only coronary thrombosis, but rheumatic and hypertensive heart disease where it is also very effective; in discovering the value of vitamin E in many diseases of the arteries in the extremities. We are proud of the considerable number of legs which should by this time be in pathological museums, but are still serving their owners in everyday life, climbing roofs, dancing, playing pipe-organs, even soldiering.

"We, of course, hope to continue our work. Our institute at London, Ontario, Canada, has more opportunity for worthwhile cardiovascular research work than any medical institution in Canada has now or has ever had. It is our constant regret that our days are filled with nothing but seeing the sick, important and merciful as that is, but we realize that this will not always be so. In the past year, we have had to turn down requests from Spanish, Indian, Syrian and German research men to join our staff since we have neither the time nor facilities for their work here.

"We have now personally treated over 8,600 cardiovascular patients [at that time—Ed.]. My great regret is that circumstances today prevent me showing you some of our hundreds of colored photographs of these people. I wonder how many people realize that this is many times the number seen in a comparable time elsewhere. We are no longer reporting on our first 10 cases. We are reporting to you on the conclusions derived from thousands. It is an investigation that Canadians and Canada should be proud of, for in this at least they lead the world.

"Everyone knows that vast sums are being raised annually by public donations and spent by the two National Heart Associations. Governments and insurance companies have likewise donated large sums to heart research. We want everyone to know that not one cent of such monies has ever been given to our work—although our investigations have been fertile in the extreme and could be so much more so with a relatively small part of this money.

"I thank you for the privilege of very briefly outlining some features of our work for you."

Comment on my part would be like gilding the lily, but I would give another suggestion to heart cases. Do not drink water that has been treated with chlorine for it uses up a portion of the body's vitamin E. I would also like to say a word on the method of making our bread. The bakers remove the wheat germ which contains vitamins B and E, iron, and other minerals. In the goodness of their hearts they enrich the bread by replacing the iron, parts of the vitamin B complex, but not a bit of the vitamin E nor the host of minerals that they so casually removed. The vitamin E that is taken out of the wheat seed goes to feed pigs and poultry. Is this crime to modern bread part of the series of reasons why we have so much heart disease?

IS THIS POSSIBLE?

In view of the overwhelming evidence that vitamin E is a most valuable aid that should long ago have been harnessed by the medical profession, it is difficult to understand why this has not been done. The puzzling attitude of the medical profession with regard to vitamin E caused *MacLeans* Magazine of Canada to make its own investigation. *MacLeans* is a long-established, conservative, and widely read magazine of large circulation. They assigned one of their best men, Eric Hutton, to do a thorough investigation and journalistic job, and his article on the subject was printed in the June 15, 1953, issue of the magazine.

Eric Hutton has done painstaking research among friends and enemies of vitamin E therapy for heart disease, has talked to physicians, members of the Heart Association of Canada, and hundreds of private individuals who are now taking vitamin E for relief of their heart or circulatory symptoms. He begins his article with the story of a Huntsville, Ontario, wholesaler, 33 of whose friends had heart attacks. Twenty of them have been treated with vitamin E and are alive. Thirteen of them who were not treated with the vitamin E are dead.

Hutton traces the story of the Shute Brothers' first interest in vitamin E to 1933, when Evan Shute, M.D., an obstetrician, used it for the treatment of habitual abortion. He discovered that it appeared to delay the normal clotting of blood. He decided to use it on a patient suffering from purpura (bleeding) who could not be operated on because of a heart condition. Treatment with vitamin E helped the heart condition more than the purpura. Dr. Shute's brother, Wilfrid, who is also an M.D., soon joined forces with Dr. Evan in treating heart and circulatory patients with their own carefully worked out vitamin E therapy.

The mother of the two Shute brothers was their next heart patient. Mrs. Shute was so ill that she was unable to walk across the room. According to her own testimony she was gardening four weeks after she began to take vitamin E. Father C. A. MacKinnon testifies for vitamin E: "Phlebitis in my legs made me a bed case. The Shutes treated me with vitamin E and now I find that I can put in an average priest's day comfortably." Mary Salmond says, "Coronary thrombosis put me on my back for four months and I was told never to work again. After vitamin E treatment I've been back on my job in a Toronto carpet plant for five years."

Shortly after the Shute brothers began to use vitamin E in the treatment of heart disease, the governing body of all physicians and surgeons practicing in Ontario summoned them to give a report on their experience with vitamin E and heart disease. They presented the report. After spending two hours deliberating over the report, while they were at lunch, the Committee decided "on evidence submitted, the committee is convinced that vitamin E has no place in the treatment of cardiovascular (heart and blood vessel) disease." Apparently their decision was based on what they call faulty diagnosis. In other words, they imply that people cured by vitamin E did not really have serious heart trouble. The Shutes answer this with the statement that in 90 per cent of the cases that come to them they do not make the first diagnosis. Patients usually come to them after seeing one, two, or three other doctors or specialists. In addition, the Shutes mention that two of the patients described in their report to the college of physicians and surgeons had been diagnosed as heart patients by physicians who were on the committee bringing in the report of incorrect diagnosis!

Asked what is their own explanation for the medical opposition to the use of vitamin E, the Shutes admit that they do not know. "Some of our loudest critics are taking vitamin E themselves. Many dispense vitamin E but will not sign a prescription for it. Many doctors returned to practice on vitamin E, after coronaries disabled them, are ashamed to admit the source of their help, even to their closest friends."

Learning recently that enough vitamin E was being shipped to a certain hospital to supply dosage for about 16 people daily, they inquired whether some special tests were under way. They were told that no hospital patients were getting vitamin E. The full supply was for the personal use of staff physicians. Recently a representative of a Windsor, Ontario, drug supply house asked Dr. Wilfrid Shute how it happened that, although London is supposed to be the world capital of vitamin E, it was not being sold in the city. Dr. Wilfrid said that of course the vitamin was being sold in every London drugstore. "Then, why is it," asked the drug supply representative, "that so many London doctors send to Windsor to have their orders filled?" The Shutes say that about 180 doctors and their families are among the 10,000 patients they have treated for heart and circulatory disease. The

Shutes, who used to be meek and mild about criticism and neglect of their methods, have decided that it is necessary for them to fight for recognition of vitamin E, regardless of whose toes are trampled on or whose feelings are hurt in the process.

Vitamin E has been the subject of extensive debate in medical magazines in the United States and abroad. Yet in Montreal a businessman, put back on his feet by the Shute treatment, decided to ask the Rotary Club to have Dr. Wilfrid Shute as a speaker. The chairman of the committee was a doctor who refused flatly to consider inviting Dr. Shute to speak. Later, when a new committee was in charge, arrangements were made for Dr. Shute to speak before the Rotary and announcements were sent out. The reaction on the part of some medical members of the Rotary was instantaneous. They protested so strongly that the committee finally agreed not to cancel the speech, but to cancel the proposed broadcast of it. Later M.D. Rotarians tried to prevent the Montreal newspaper from publishing accounts of the speech. Mr. McConnell, the publisher of the *Montreal Star,* and members of his staff had benefited from being treated with vitamin E. So, in addition to defending freedom of the press, the *Star* editorial board was defending a friend whose integrity was unquestioned, when they published the following editorial:

"Montreal's reputation as a hospitable, courteous and open-minded city suffered, we fear, some damage as a result of the controversy inside the Rotary Club, and now outside of it as well, over the speech made this week by Dr. Wilfrid Shute. It is not a suitable thing—putting the case mildly—to invite a reputable man to Montreal to make a speech and then to take such steps as can be taken to restrict his audience and subject him to discourtesy. Far better to cancel the invitation altogether.

"Dr. Shute's address was on the use of vitamin E in the treatment of heart disease. This is a topic of great medical controversy, one upon which there are legitimate differences of opinion. But for some lamentable reason certain medical men feel so strongly that they are prepared to go to great length to prevent public discussion of it. This is not only unscientific, it also does no credit to a great and honorable profession which has done so much to push back the frontiers of medical knowledge. The advocates of the treatment in question are neither quacks nor charlatans and in a free society, they are entitled to have their say.

"The Shute incident here is, unfortunately, not an isolated one in the record and history of medicine. Again and again the restless and enquiring mind has suffered slights and indignities at the hands of men who have refused to open new doors or even to walk through them when they have been opened by others."

In a survey done by Mr. Hutton among pharmaceutical houses which prepare vitamin E, he was told that in Toronto 28 per cent of the doctors use vitamin E and approve of its therapy, even though they will not indicate openly their approval. In a survey made by one company among 800 doctor customers, 228 made enthusiastic comments on the effectiveness of vitamin E in treating heart disease. Mr. Hutton goes on: "I spoke to an eminent physicist, a man largely responsible for a major Canadian contribution to the secret armament of World War II. He had personally found in vitamin E such a source of physical and mental endurance and efficiency that he had expressed the opinion that in a close war vitamin E supplied to key personnel might actually make the difference between victory and defeat. I asked him if he would tell his story. He thought the matter over and then replied: 'No, I would like to, because it is truly remarkable. But somehow the medical profession has managed to give the idea that anyone who believes in vitamin E is—well, slightly in the screwball class. I just don't feel that I should expose myself to the inevitable comments if I speak openly.' "

I think it is more than that. If you take the heart cases out of doctors' offices (and the taking of vitamin E poses a threat of it) more than half the income of the medical profession will vanish. A heart disease case is an annuity for the doctors, and people will continue to die because they are caught in the toils of economics—mink coats for doctors' wives, Cadillacs, and stock and bond investments. This state of affairs will continue as long as the medical profession is permitted to police itself.

Spare the rod and spoil the child. We must adopt a "get tough" program with the medical profession. I suggest the appointment of a national group comprised of engineers, businessmen, and suchlike folk to make an independent investigation of this regrettable vitamin E scandal.

Appendix C

Analysis and Comments by Dr. E.V. Shute on Some Unfavorable Reports on Vitamin E Therapy

VITAMIN E THERAPY CRITICIZED

INTRODUCTION

Very soon after our initial publications on our discovery fifteen papers appeared in English language journals which contradicted our findings on the value of alpha tocopherol in cardiovascular diseases. Three of these papers were duplicates, published in alternative journals; there really were twelve papers, therefore. I will consider all of these briefly in order.

MAKINSON, OLEESKY AND STONE (ENGLAND)—LANCET, 1:102, 1948

Their study reported 22 cases of angina. None of them had had a coronary thrombosis in the previous six months. Each was given 150 mgm of synthetic alpha tocopherol for three weeks' trial. Ten of these were helped, but they point out that a corresponding number were helped with phenobarbital, a mere sedative.

Comment: The dose here is no more than half of the dose we had suggested. We always have contended that a dose at this level is completely inadequate for anginas or coronaries of any kind. The trial was *very* brief; even at that these workers reported that almost 50% were helped and that would recommend almost any treatment for angina, which is notoriously difficult to treat. Curiously enough, shortly after this the Department of Surgery of the same University (University of Manchester) came out with studies showing how effective alpha tocopherol was in the treatment of intermittent claudication, a kind of angina in the leg brought on by arteriosclerosis of the vessels there. How a substance can be good for arteriosclerosis of the leg and be useless for arteriosclerosis of the vessels of the heart, which is the common cause of angina, and how two adjacent departments of the same hospital can disagree so completely, is hard to imagine.

BALL (ENGLAND) LANCET, 1:116, 1948

10 patients with moderate or severe angina. 5 were hypertensive and 4 had had coronary thrombosis. Each was given 300 mgm synthetic alpha tocopherol for six weeks or more. Two were helped markedly or moderately.

Comment: This author points out that Evans and Hoyle have shown that placebos alone should regularly help 40%. This means, of course, that even an inert substance should help 40% of anginas, whereas in this series only 20% were helped. There must therefore be something wrong with the arrangement of the experiment, or with the observations. Surely, alpha tocopherol must be at least as good as a placebo.

LEVY AND BOAS (U.S.A.)—ANNALS OF INTERNAL MEDICINE, 28:1117, 1948

These authors treated 13 cases. 5 were chronic anginas, 3 were acute anginas, 5 were patients with chronic heart failure. They were given 200 to 800 mgm daily of alpha tocopherol. All patients with chronic heart failure were given large doses up to 600 mgm daily, which, as we have repeatedly warned, is enough to throw all of them into even worse heart failure. We have long stressed the danger of overdosage in just this group of cases. No improvement at all was noted.

Comment: Here again, even an inert placebo should have improved at least 40% of these anginas. These findings throw doubt on the validity of the whole experiment.

BAER, HEINE AND GELFOND (U.S.A.)—AMERICAN JOURNAL OF MEDICAL SCIENCES, 215:542, 1948

BAER, HEINE AND GELFOND (U.S.A.)—MODERN CONCEPTS OF CARDIOVASCULAR DISEASE, 18:57, 1949

BAER, HEINE AND GELFOND (U.S.A.)—ANNALS NEW YORK ACADEMY OF SCIENCES, 52:412, 1949

These authors treated 22 cases—11 were in congestive failure and 5 were anginas, 6 were hypertensive and/or arteriosclerotic. The patients were given 300 to 400 mgm synthetic alpha tocopherol daily. Of the 11 in failure 3 were questionably helped. Of the anginas none were helped. Of the hypertensives none were helped.

Comment: Same as before. The congestive failures never should have had such a high dose. We have repeatedly warned against it. If the experiment had been properly set up and properly observed, alpha tocopherol should have done at least as well on the anginas and the hypertensives as placebos. Placebos should have helped at least 40%.

RAVEN AND KATZ (U.S.A.)—NEW ENGLAND JOURNAL OF MEDICINE, 240:331, 1949

11 anginas were treated with 250 mgm alpha tocopherol daily. 2 were slightly helped over a period of 4 to 24 weeks.

Comment: The dose is much too small for anginas. The number of these that should have been helped by an inert placebo was more than 2.

DONEGAN, MESSER, ORGAIN AND RUFFIN (U.S.A.)—AMERICAN
JOURNAL OF MEDICAL SCIENCES, 217:294, 1949

7 hypertensives, 7 hypertensives with hypertrophy and 7
anginas were given 75 to 600 mgm alpha tocopherol daily.
The duration of the study is not stated. Two of the 7 hypertensives were helped, none of the hypertensives with hypertrophy, and one of the 7 anginas.

Comment: Here again an inert substance should have done
better and this casts doubt on the validity of the conclusions.

BAUM AND STEIN (U.S.A.)—WISCONSIN MEDICAL JOURNAL,
48:315, 1949

200 to 600 mgm alpha tocopherol were given for 9 to 155
days to 13 anginas and 17 patients in failure. 4 of these patients got improvement in vital capacity of 500 c.c. or greater,
2 of the 12 hypertensives had a fall of blood pressure, but
both showed increasing failure. Of the 13 anginas 8% were
moderately improved and 15% were slightly improved, making
an improvement rate of 23%. Of the 17 patients in failure
18% were improved, one developed a great diuresis and 1
showed much less dyspnoea. 3 patients with fibrillation showed
no change.

Comment: as before.

RINZLER, BAKST, BENJAMIN, BOBB AND TRAVELL (U.S.A.)—
ANNALS NEW YORK ACADEMY OF SCIENCES, 52:345,
1949

RINZLER, BAKST, BENJAMIN, BOBB AND TRAVELL (U.S.A.)—
CIRCULATION, 1:288, 1950

29 cases of chest pain some being anginas and some not,
14 of these being controls and treated with placebos. They
were given 200 to 300 mgm alpha tocopherol for an average
of 10 to 20 weeks. In the patients with chest pain the placebos
cured 27% and the alpha tocopherol 37%. In the anginas

placebos cured 22% and alpha tocopherol 33%. 14% of these got worse when taking placebos, but none got worse when taking alpha tocopherol. In non-anginal chest pain 40% were helped by placebos, 50% by alpha tocopherol.

Comment: This illustrates again what placebos should be able to do. They should cure about 40% of all patients having pain. It is amazing, therefore, that alpha tocopherol and placebos didn't do this well with angina, although alpha tocopherol always did better than the placebos. The dose here was probably too small to show what alpha tocopherol could really do.

RUSH (U.S.A.)—CALIFORNIA MEDICINE, 71:391, 1949

12 anginas, 22 anginas with sclerosis, and 22 patients with angina following coronary thrombosis were treated with vitamin E. There was subjective help in 3 of the first group, 2 of the second and 2 of the third, all of which could be duplicated with placebos.

Comment: Here again the results with alpha tocopherol aren't good enough, even if alpha tocopherol were only a placebo, and this challenges the validity of the experiment.

EISEN AND GROSS (U.S.A.)—NEW YORK STATE JOURNAL OF MEDICINE, 49:2422, 1949

These authors treated 16 cases of arteriosclerotic heart disease, 5 cases of arteriosclerotic heart disease with congestive failure, 1 case of hypertensive heart disease, 2 cases of chronic rheumatic heart disease with failure, 12 peripheral arteriosclerotics and 2 cases of Buerger's disease. The patients were given 150 to 800 mgm of a poor preparation of vitamin E every day for two to twelve months. This contained at the most 75 to 400 mgm of alpha tocopherol. No benefit was received in any of these cases.

Comment: Here is an obviously biased conclusion. In this study alpha tocopherol has no placebo value of any kind. This result is particularly striking as scores of authors since have found that this substance was useful for peripheral arteriosclerosis in carefully controlled experiments and also there have been fine results in cases of Buerger's disease so treated. This experiment obviously should be thrown out of court as indicating gross bias.

LEMLEY, GALE, FURMAN, CHERRINGTON, DERBY AND MENEELY (U.S.A.)—AMERICAN HEART JOURNAL, 39:1029, 1949

Alpha tocopherol is of no value at all in heart disease because studies of plasma tocopherol showed that its level was unrelated to any heart phenomena.

Comment: This study was based on the idea that tocopherol deficiency is causally related to heart disease and therefore the correction of that deficiency should relieve the heart disease. We have repeatedly stated we use alpha tocopherol as a pharmacodynamic agent per se, and our dose is not related to its use as a vitamin. We use it as we would any other pharmacological agent. These findings are therefore irrelevant to our observations.

EICHERT (U.S.A.)—SOUTHERN MEDICAL JOURNAL, 42:717, 1949

19 patients were given 200 to 300 mgm alpha tocopherol daily for 3 weeks to 4 months. These included 4 arteriosclerotics, 6 coronaries, 3 hypertensives, 2 rheumatics and 4 cases of peripheral vascular disease. There was no change in the arteriosclerotics, 3 of the 6 coronaries were moderately helped. No improvement in the hypertensives and no improvement in the 2 rheumatics. 1 of the 4 peripheral vasculars was helped. There were 3 deaths in all.

Comment: The dosage here was too small in all the cases treated except the rheumatic hearts. These were certainly overdosed. The observations on peripheral vascular disease are contradicted by scores of workers who have published since this time. It is interesting that 50% of his coronary cases were helped. Most of this experiment appears to be irrelevant.

General Observations

Nearly all of these studies were done before the value of placebos was realized by clinical experimenters. The result is that they betray their bias or malice so often in their conclusions by finding alpha tocopherol "useless" or "completely valueless." Nothing can be therapeutically valueless, it is now known, especially where pain is the criterion, as in angina. Placebos are therapy in themselves. Alpha tocopherol *must* have helped 40% of all anginas treated. To find less throws out the whole study. . . .

Bibliography

ACCORNERO, S. R. (Italy) *Proc. 3rd Internat. Cong. on Vit. E,* Venice, Italy, p. 452, Sept. 1955.

AITKEN, F. C., AND HYTTEN, F. E. (Scotland): "Infant Feeding: Comparison of Breast and Artificial Feeding." *Nutrition Abstr. & Revs.,* 30:341, 1960.

ANISIMOV, V. E. (U.S.S.R.) *Klinicheskaia Meditsina,* 36:147–8, 1958.

ASLAN, A. (Munich) "Geriatrics in Rumania," *Med. Klin.,* 52:1758, 1957

ASTRAND, P. O. (U.S.A.) *Physiological Reviews,* 36:307, 1956.

BACIGALUPO, F. A., CULIK, R., LUECKE, R. W., THORP, F., JR., AND JOHNSTON, R. L. (U.S.A.) "Further Studies on Vitamin E Deficiency in the Lamb." *J. An. Sci.,* 11:609, 1952.

BAILEY, HERBERT "He Died That Others May Live." *Pageant,* Aug. 1951.

BARWICK-SCHRAMM, A., AND DUMANSKA, K. (Warsaw) "The Effect of Vitamin E on Aldolase Activity in Rheumatoid Arthritis." *Polskie Arch. Med. Wewnetrznej,* 29:35, 1959.

BARWICK-SCHRAMM, A., AND MOL, A. (Warsaw) "The Effect of Vitamin E on the Efficiency of Skeletal Muscle and the General State of Patients Suffering from Chronic Progressive Polyarthritis." *Fysiat. Vestnik,* 35:281, 1957.

BAUER, W. W. *Your Health Today,* Harper Brothers, N.Y., 1955.

BAUR, L. S. "Principles of Artificial Infant Feeding." *J. Am. Pharm. Assoc., Pract. Pharm. Ed.,* 16:96, 1955.

BAYER, R. (Germany) "Results of Pretreatment with Vitamin E for Control of Primary and Secondary Essential Infertility; Reports on Studies with 100 Married Couples." *Wien. med. Wochschr.,* 109:271, 1959.

BECKER-FREYSANG, H. (Germany) *Arch. f. exp. Path. u. Pharmak.,* 214:411, 1952.

BECKMAN, R. (Germany) "Vitamin E, Choline and Inositol for Muscle Disorders." *Munch. med. Woch.,* 94:1176, 1952.

BECKMAN, R. (Germany) "Results of Experiments on the Vitamin E Content of Human Milk and of Cow's Milk and its Use in Pediatrics." *Milchwissenschaft*, 9:365, 1954.

———— "The Vitamin E Content of Milk." *Medizinsche*, p. 1638, 1954.

———— "Observations on the Metabolism and Therapy of Primary Myopathies, Especially Erb's Progressive Muscular Dystrophy." *Medizinische*, 50:1771 and 52:1847, 1956.

———— "Vitamin E in Pediatrics." *Arch. Kinderheilk*, 157:7, 1958.

———— "Carbohydrate metabolism; the Activity of Fructose-1, 6-Diphosphate Aldolase in Serum and Functionally Limited Changes in Liver Growth in the Newborn and Young Infant." *Monatsschr. Kinderheilk*, 107:258, 1959.

———— "Present Status of the Therapy of Erb's Progressive Muscular Dystrophy." *Arch. Kinderheilk*, 159:217, 1959.

———— "The Artificial Feeding of Well and Sick Infants." *Tagl. Praxis*, 1:87, 1960.

BELLOTTI, R., RAVERA, M., AND ABBONA, C. *Arch. e Maragli di Patol. e Clinica*, 9:529, 1954.

BENSON, T. F. (New York State Vet. College, Ithaca, N.Y.) "New Insight into Causes and Effective Treatment of Mink Diseases." *The Black Fox Magazine and Modern Mink Breeder*, 42(12):8–10, 19, April, 1959.

BERGEL, M. (Argentina) "Pathogenesis of Leprosy." *La Semana Med.*, 109:3, 1956.

BISHOP, E. H., AND WOUTERSZ, T. B. (U.S.A.) "Arrest of Premature Labour." *J.A.M.A.*, 178:812, 1961.

BLANK, B. "Further results of our Method of Treatment of Recently Born Premature Babies and of Feeble Babies." *Dia. Med.*, 26:958, 1954.

BLOCK, M. T. (U.S.A.) "Vitamin E in the Treatment of Diseases of the Skin." *Clin. Med.*, 60:1, 1953.

BOCK, R. F. "Alpha Tocopherol in Gynecological Practice; a 12-Year Clinical Evaluation." *Ariz. Med.*, 16:100, 1959.

BONADONNA, T., AND KAAN, I. (Italy) "First Results of the Administration of Vitamin A and Vitamin E to Bulls." *Zootec. e vet.*, 9:148, 1954.

BONFERT, A., AND ARP, J. "Contribution on the Use of Vitamin E Preparations in Certain Cases of Sterility in Cattle." *Tierarztl. Umschau*, 8:455, 1953.

BONOMINI, V. (Italy) "On the Synergism of Cocarboxylase-Sulfur-Tocopherol in Treatment of Hepatic Parenchymal Insufficiency." *Clin. Terap.*, 13:528, 1957.

BOOTH, V. H., AND HOBSON-FROHOCK, A. J. (England): "Alpha Tocopherol Content of Leaves as Affected by Growth Rate." *J. Sci. of Food and Agric.*, 3:251, 1961.

BORY, R., AND CAPLIER, P. (France) "Treatment of Vulvar Pruritis." *Gaz. med. France*, 65:1321, 1958.

BOYER, R. (Austria) "Vitamin E in Habitual Abortion." *Geburts. u frauenheil.*, 16:394, 1956.

BRAUNSTEIN, H. (U.S.A.) "Tocopherol Deficiency in Adults with Chronic Pancreatitis." *Gastroenterology*, 40:224, 1961.

British Medical Journal "Vitamin E Therapy," 1960:1905.

BROWN, A. M., COOK, M. J., LANE-PETTER, W., PORTER, G., AND TUFFERY, A. A. (England) "Influence of Nutrition on Reproduction in Laboratory Rodents." *Proc. Nutrition Soc.*, 19:32, 1960.

BUCHNER, F. (Germany) "Congenital Anomalies." *German Medical Monthly*, 1:261, 1956.

BURCH, G. E., AND DE PASQUALE, N. P. (U.S.A.) "Haematocrit, Blood Viscosity and Myocardial Infarction" (editorial). *Amer. J. Medicine*, 32:161, 1962.

BUTTURINI, U. *Giorn. Clin. Med.*, 22:4, 1941.

——— *Giorn. Clin. Med.*, 22:14, 1941.

——— *Pathologia*, 33:602, 1942.

——— *Klin. Woch.*, 21:609, 1942.

——— *L'Ateneo Parmense*, 15:5, 1943–44.

——— *Giorn. Clin. Med.*, 26:7, 1945.

——— *Ann. N.Y. Acad. Science*, 52:397, 1949.

——— *Min. Medica*, 49:11, 1950.

——— *Giorn. Clin. Med.*, 31:1, 1950.

——— *Journ. Therapeut. de Paris*, p. 331, Ed. Doin, 1950.

——— *Il Diabete da Allossana*. Ed. Min. Medica, Torino, 1951.

——— *La Clin. Terapeut.*, 2:31, 1952.

——— *Proc. 3rd Internat. Cong. Vit. E*, Venice, Italy, p. 46, Sept. 1955.

BUTTURINI, U., AND BAGNI, L. *Giorn Clin. Med.*, 23:6, 1942.

BUTTURNI, U., AND BARONCHELLI, A. *Boll. Soc. Ital. Biol. Sperim.*, 26:5, 1950.

——— *Gior. di Clin. Med.*, 32:552, 1951.

BUTTURINI, U., AND VOLTA, M. *Boll. Soc. Ital. Biol. Sperim.*, 26:5, 1950.

——— *Rass. Fisiop. Clin. e Terap.*, 22:8, 1950.

CANESTRI, G., AND PICCOTTI, M. L. (Italy) "Concentrations of Vitamin E in the Blood of the Infant." *Minerva Pediat.*, 13:592, 1961.

CANTIN, M., DIEUDONNE, JEAN-MARIE, AND SELYE, H. (Canada) "Effects of Vitamin E on Cardiomuscular Calciphylactic Lesions." *Exp. Med. and Surg.*, 318:20, 1962.

CASTELAR PINHEIRO, G., DA ROCHA CASTELAR PINHEIRA, R. M. V., AND DALCORSO FILHO, P. "Progressive Muscular Dystrophy." *Arch. bras. med.*, 49:137, 1959.

CATELLA, H. (France) "Use of Alpha Tocopherol Quinone in Hypertension." *Praxis*, 38:988, 1961.

CERVELLATI, L., AND MASSEI, M. (Italy) "Serum Levels of Vitamin E in Normal and Toxic Pregnancies in the Puerperium." *Acta Vitamin*, 4:197, 1950.

CHENG, D. W., AND THOMAS, B. H. (U.S.A.) "Histological Changes in the Abnormal Rat Foetuses Induced by Maternal Vitamin E Deficiency." *Anat. Record*, 121:274, 1955.

CHOUDBURY, A. K. R., AND NANDI, R. N. (India) *Calcutta M. J.*, 53:414, 1956.

CLEIN, L. J., WILLIAMS, H. T. G., AND MACBETH, R. A. (Canada) "The Use of Alpha Tocopherol in the Treatment of Intermittent Claudication." *C.M.A.J.*, 86:215, 1962.

CLEMENT, R. (France) "Spontaneous Atherosclerosis in Wild Animals." *Presse Med.*, 69:2478, 1961.

COMI, G., AND NESI, G. (Italy) *Riv. Crit. di Clin. Med.*, 50:214, 1950.

CONSTANTINI, A., AND RICCI, C. (Italy) "Influence of Alpha Tocopherol and Calcium Gluconate on Blood Coagulation." *Chir. gen.*, 1:300, 1951.

CROSS, R. F. (Ireland) "Prevention of Anencephaly and Foetal Abnormalities by a Preconception Regimen." *Lancet*, 2:1124, 1961.

CROSSE, V. M. "Vitamin E and Hyaline Membranes." *IX Intern. Congr. of Pediatrics*, July 19–25, 1959, Montreal, Can., p. 59; Medizinische 1960, 11.

CULIK, R., BACIGALUPO, F. A., THORP, F., LUECKE, R. W., AND NELSON, R. H. (U.S.A.) *J. Animal Science*, 10:1006, 1951.

"Current Estimates from the Health Interview Survey, July 1962– June 1963" Washington, D.C.: U.S. Dept. of Health, Education, and Welfare, 1964.

CURTO, G. M. (Italy) *Zootec. Vet.*, 12:203, 1957.

D'AGOSTINO BARBARO, A. (Italy) "Organotropic Activity of Vitamin E; Histologic Research." *Riv. zootec.*, 24:1, 1951.

DALLA TORRE, L., AND BOLDRINI, R. (Italy) *Clinica Nuova*, 12:617, 1952.

DALLE COSTE, P., AND KLINGER, R. (Italy) "Alpha Tocopherol in Diabetic Diseases of the Veins." *Riforma Med.*, 69:853, 1955.

DARLINGTON, F. G., AND CHASSELS, J. B. (Canada) "A Further Study of the Breeding and Racing of Thoroughbred Horses Given Large Doses of Alpha Tocopherol." *Summary*, 12:55, 1956.

———— "Alpha Tocopherol and the Breeding of Thoroughbred Horses." *Summary*, 10:66, 1958.

———— "Final, Inclusive Report on Five-Year Study on the Effect of Administering Alpha Tocopherol to Thoroughbreds." *Summary*, 12:52, 1960.

DA RUGNA, D. (Switz.) "Experience with the Conservative Treatment of Impaired Sperm Formation in Sterility. Effects of Different Types of Treatment on Fertility." *Schweiz. med. Wochschr.*, 88:563, 597, 1958.

DATTA, A. K. (India) "An Appraisal of the Function of Vitamin E." *Indian Practitioner*, 11:523, 1958.

DAVIDIAN, H. (Iran) "Treatment of Opium Addicts with Vitamin E." *Acta Med. Iran*, 1:215, 1956–1957.

DE CAMPOS MAGALHAES, M. J., AND FIGUEIREDO BARBOSA, A. J. "Treatment of Amyotrophy of the Hands of Leprous Patients with Local Injections of Vitamin E." *Medico* (Porto), 9:97, 1958.

DE CARLO, M., ZINOLLI, L., AND CASERTANO, F. (Italy) "Contribution to the Study of Climacteric Muscular Dystrophy." *Arch. "E Maragliano" patol. e clin.*, 14:707, 1958.

DEL GIUDICE, A. (Buenos Aires) "Massive Doses of Vitamin E as a Factor in Mental Improvement." *Dia. Med.*, 29:1814, 1957.

———— "Large Doses of Vitamin E as a Factor in the Mental Improvement of Subnormal Children." *Summary*, 12:21, 1960; *Semana med.*, 116:46, 1960.

DELINOTTE, B. A. C., AND VONTHRON, A. "Medical Treatment of Urinary Incontinence with Vitamin E." *Gaz. med. France*, 67:171, 1960.

DERITTER, E., MAGID, L., AND SLEEZER, P. E. (U.S.A.) "Vitamins in Cosmetics." *Am. Perfumer*, 73:54, 1959.

DESUSCLADE, C., AND DESUSCLADE, D. "Evolutive Myopia. Pathogenesis and Treatment with Vitamin E." *Presse Med.*, 67:855, 1959.

DI FIORE, V., AND AICARDI, G. (Italy) "Action of Alpha Tocopherol on Climacteric." *Quaderni di Clin. Obstet. e Ginic.*, 7:31, 1952.

DI LEO, P., AND CECILIANI, L. (Italy) "Osteogenesis in Prolonged Avitaminosis E." *Boll. Soc. Ital. Biol. Sper.*, 37:402, 1961.

DINDA, M. M. (India) *Indian Med. Forum*, 4:361, 1953.

EMMEL, V. M. (U.S.A.) "Kidney Changes in Vitamin E Deficiency." *J. Nutrition*, 61:51, 1957.

ENGLARO, G. C., AND VIDAL, B. (Italy) "Treatment of Induratio Penis Plastica (Peyronie's Disease)." *Friuli med.*, 12:259, 1957.

EVANS, H. M., BISHOP, K. S. *J. Metab. Res.*, 3:233, 1923.

Exercise and Fitness, The Athletic Institute, 1959.

FAJER, A., CARNEIRO, H. B., AND ORIA, H. (Brazil) "Effect of Vitamin E on the Incidence of Gastric Ulcers in Rats on Simplified Diets." *Hospital*, 48:543, 1955.

FALCON, J. H. "Sclerema of the Newborn." *Semana med.*, 106:935, 1955.

FANG, H. S., HALL, A. L., AND HWANG, T. F. "Combined Effects of Vitamins A and E on Dark Adaptation in Man." *Am. J. Optom.*, 37:93, 1960.

FAULKNER, J. A. (U.S.A.) "Physical Activity, Health and Longevity." *Summary*, 14:1, 1962.

FERES, G., AND BANGE, C. (France) "Comparative Study of the Metabolic Effects of Tocopherol and Alpha Tocopherol Quinone." *Rev. de Path. Generale et de Physiol. Clinique*, 61:183, 1961.

FERNANDEZ, M. (Italy) "Use of Testosterone and Vitamin E in Cure of Prostatic Hypertrophy." *Arch. Ital. de Urologia*, 24:442, 1951.

FINLAYSON, R., AND SYMONS, C. S. (England) "Arterial Disease in Man and Animals." *New Scientist*, 12:470, 1961.

———— "Arteriosclerosis in Wild Animals in Captivity." *Proc. R. S. of Med.*, 973:54, 1961.

FISHER, B., DEBAKEY, M. E., AND MOSES, C. (U.S.A.) "Peripheral Arterial Diseases." *Postgrad. Med.*, 30:374, 1961.

FLOCH, H., AND HORTH, R. (Fr. Guinea) "Vitamin E Therapy in Neuritis and Trophic Disturbances of Leprosy." *Boll. Soc. Path. Exot.*, 45:157, 1952.

FREY, I. G. (Germany) "Combination of Short Waves and Vitamin E for Late Roentgen Damage to Skin." *Strahlentherapie*, 95:440, 1954.

FREY, J. (Germany) *Arch. f. exp. Path. u. Pharmakol.*, 221:466–476, 1954.

FURUHJELM, M., JONSON, B., AND LAGERGREN, C. G. (Sweden) "Quality of Human Semen in Spontaneous Abortion." *Internat. J. of Fertility*, 7:17, 1962.

GAMALERO, P. C. (Italy) "Influence of Vitamin E on the Blood Lipid Pattern in Infancy." *Minerva Pediat.*, 10:1342, 1958.

Garetta (France) Thesis: "Vitamin E for Leg Ulcers." *Toulouse*, #91, 1949.

GEISENDORF, M. W. "Treatment of Pre-Menstrual Syndrome with Vitamins A and E." *Bull. Federation soc. gynecol. et obstet. langue franc.*, 10:3, 1958.

GENTILI, C., AND CORSI, A. (Italy) "Clinical and Histological Features of Menopausal Muscular Dystrophy." *Minerva med.*, 51:2757, 1960.

GERLOCZY, F. (Hungary) "Sclerodema of Premature Infants, a Deficiency Disease." *Paediat. danub.*, 5:169, 1949.

———— "The Importance of Vitamin E in Pediatrics." *Orvosi Hetilap*, 45:1606, 1959.

———— "Vitamin E Deficiency States in Newborn and Nursing Infants." *IX Intern. Congr. of Pediatrics*, July 19–25, 1959, Montreal, Can., p. 73.

GERLOCZY, F., AND BENCZE, B. (Hungary) "New Studies on Vitamin E Deficiency in the Newborn and Their Nutrition." *Acta Paediat. Hung.*, 1:35, 1960.

GERLOCZY, F., BENCZE, B., AND IVANYI, K. (Hungary) "Vitamin E in the Vernix Caseosa." *Zeits f. Vitaminforsch*, 1961.

GERLOCZY, F., BENCZE, B., AND KASSAI, S. (Hungary) "High Dosage of Natural Vitamin E in the Treatment of Acute Thrombophlebitis During Infancy and Chronic Thrombophlebitis in Adults." Read at *Fourth International Conference on Vitaminology*, Sofia, Bulgaria, 1960.

GERLOCZY, F., BENCZE, B., KASSAI, S., AND BARTA, L. (Hungary) "The Vasoprotective Role of Vitamin E in Children, also a Note on Diabetic Necrobiosis." *Gyermekgyogyaszat*, 12:225, 1961.

GERLOCZY, F., BENCZE, B., MALIK, T., AND UGRAY, M. (Hungary) "Vitamin Metabolism in Infantile Atrophy." *Acta Med. Acad. Sci. Hung.*, 12:1, 1958.

———— "Vitamin E Content of the Blood Plasma in Cases of Infantile Atrophy." *Annales Paediatrici*, 192:20, 1959.

GERSHOFF, S. N., AND NORKIN, S. A. (U.S.A.) "Vitamin E Deficiency in Cats." *J. Nutrition*, 77:303, 1962.

GERVASONI, A. AND VANNOTTI, A. (Switzerland) "Vitamin E and Arteriosclerosis." *Schweiz. Med. Woch.*, 86:708, 1956.

GIMLETTE, T. M. D. (England) "The Muscular Lesion in Hyperthyroidism." *Brit. Med. J.*, 1959, 1143.

GLAUNER, W. (Germany) "Hypotensive Action of Vitamin E in Essential Hypertension." *Deutsche. Med. Woch.*, 77:627, 1952.

GOODHART, R. S. (U.S.A.) "Rational Use of Vitamins in the Practice of Medicine." *Postgrad. Med.*, 27:663, 1960.

GORBAN, M. G., AND KRAMER, M. (Hungary) "Blood Levels of Vitamin E in Habitual Abortion." *C. R. de Soc. Franc. de Gynecologie*, 26:65, 1956.

GORDIN, R., KOSKENOJA, M., LAMBERG, B. A., LINDQVIST, C., OLIN-LAMBERG, C., AND PIHKANEN, T. (Finland) "Myotonic Dystrophy." *Acta. Med. Scand.*, 166:151, 1960.

GORDON, H. H., NITOWSKY, H. M., AND CORNBLATH, M. (U.S.A.) "Studies of Tocopherol Deficiency in Infants and Children." *A.M.A. J. Diseases Children*, 90:669, 1955.

GORDON, H. H., NITOWSKY, H. M., AND TILDON, J. T. (U.S.A.) "Tocopherol Deficiency in Infants and Children with Steatorrhea." *Trans. Am. Clin. Climatol. Assoc.*, 68:155, 1956; *IX Intern. Cong. Paediatrics*, July 19, 1959, p. 118 (Montreal, Canada).

GORDON, H. H., NITOWSKY, H. M., TILDON, J. T., AND LEVIN, S. "Studies of Tocopherol Deficiency in Infants and Children." *Pediatrics*, 21:673, 1958.

GORIA, A. (Italy) *Boll. della Soc. Ital. di Biol. Sper.*, 29:1275, 1277, 1953.

GORIA, A., AND MALLEN, J. (Italy) *Ibid.*, 29:1278, 1953.

GRABOWSKI, C. T. (U.S.A.) "Hypoxia and Chick Embryo Anomalies." *Am. J. Anat.*, 109:25, 1961.

GRANJON, A., YANNOTTI, S., AND CEDARD, L. (France) "Blood Levels of Oestrogen in Fibroids." *Presse Med.*, 69:2191, 1961.

GRAY, D. E. (Hong Kong) *J. of Vitaminology*, 4:122, 1958.

GROS, H., AND KIRNBERGER, E. J. (Germany) "Vitamin E for Erb's Progressive Muscular Dystrophy." *Klin. Woch.*, 30:780, 1950.

GRUBB, E. (Sweden) "Tocopherols for Skin Diseases." *Acta Dermato-Venereol.*, 32:256, 1952.

GUHRKE, K-H. "Experiences with Vitamin E in the Local Treatment of Parodontopathies." *Deut. Stomatol.*, 6:495, 1956.

HADNAGY, C., KELEMEN, L., MOZES, M., SZILAGYI, D., LASZLO, L., RAVASZ, J., PALENESAR, A., AND ZSEMLYEI, L. M. (Romania) "The Action of Vitamin E on the Intermediary Carbohydrate Metabolism in Acute Hepatitis." *Deutsch Zeits f. Verdauungs u. Stoffwechselkrank.*, 21:138, 1961.

HAIMOVICI, H. (U.S.A.) "Peripheral Arterial Disease in Diabetes." *N.Y. State J. of Med.*, 61:2988, 1961.

HARMAN, D. (U.S.A.) "Atherosclerosis: Possible Ill-Effects of the Use of Highly Unsaturated Fats to Lower Serum-Cholesterol Levels." *Lancet*, 11:1116, 1957.

HARRIS, P. L., HARDENBROOK, E. G., DEAN, F. P., CUSACK, E. R., AND JENSEN, J. L. (U.S.A.) "Blood Tocopherol Values in Normal Human Adults and Incidence of Vitamin E Deficiency." *Proc. of Soc. for Exp. Biol. and Med.*, 107:381, 1961.

HARTROFT, W. S., AND O'NEAL, R. B. (U.S.A.) "Experimental Coronary Atherosclerosis." *Amer. J. Cardiology*, 9:355, 1962.

Health and Fitness in the Modern World, The Athletic Institute, 1961.

"Health Statistics from the U.S. National Health Survey: Chronic Conditions Causing Limitation of Activities, July 1959–June 1961." Washington, D.C.: U.S. Dept. of Health, Education, and Welfare, 1962.

HILLMAN, R. W. (U.S.A.) "Tocopherol Excess in Man Creatinuria Associated with Prolonged Ingestion." *Am. J. Nutrition*, 5:597, 1957.

HIRSCH, S. (U.S.A.) "Clinical Observations on Migraine and Its Treatment." *N.Y. State J. of Medicine*, 54:5, Mar. 1, 1954.

——— "The 'Well' Patient Who Feels Sick." *N.Y. State J. of Medicine*, 55:8, Apr. 15, 1955.

HORNE, H. W., JR., AND MADDOCK, C. L. (U.S.A.) "Vitamin A Therapy in Oligospermia." *Fertility and Sterility*, 3:245, 1952.

HORWITT, M. K. (U.S.A.) "Tocopherol Requirements of Man." *Federation Proc.*, 18:530, 1959.

——— "Vitamin E and Lipid Metabolism in Man." *Am. J. Clin. Nutrition*, 8:451, 1960.

HORWITT, M. K., AND BAILEY, P. (U.S.A.) "Cerebellar Pathology in an Infant Resembling Chick Nutritional Encephalomalacia." *A.M.A. Arch. Neurol.*, 1:312, 1959.

HORWITT, M. K., HARVEY, C. C., CENTURY, B., AND WITTING, L. A. (U.S.A.) "Polyunsaturated Lipids and Tocopherol Requirements." *J. Am. Dietetic Assoc.*, 38:231, 1961.

HORWITT, M. K., HARVEY, C. C., AND MEYER, B. J. (U.S.A.) "Plasma Tocopherol, Hemolysis and Dietary Unsaturated Lipid Relationships in Man." *Federation Proc.*, 17:245, 1958.

HOUCHIN, D. B., MATTILL, H. A. (U.S.A.) *J. Biol. Chem.*, 146:301, 1942.

HOULE, G. R. (U.S.A.) "Vitamin E Deficiency in Beef Cattle." *J. Am. Vet. Med. Assoc.*, 121:485, 1952.

HOVE, E. D., HICKMAN, K., HARRIS, P. L. *Arch. Biochem.*, 8:395, 1945.

HUGHES, E. C. (U.S.A.) "Preconceptional Approach to Prevention of Early Foetal Death." *Clin. Obst. & Gyn.,* 4:402, 1961.

HUNTER, J. D. (New Zealand) "Cholesterol Levels in Polynesians." *Fed. Proc.,* 21 (Part 2) 76, 1962.

ITO, Z. (Japan) "Stress Creatinuria and Vitamin E." *Nippon Seirigaku Zasshi,* 22:321, 1960 (see *Chem. Abst.,* 55:1937, 1961).

JACQUES, W. H. (Canada) "Vitamin E in Chronic Poliomyelitis." *Can. Med. Assoc. J.,* 81:129, 1959.

JAVERT, C. T. (U.S.A.) "Prevention of Habitual Abortion." *Bull. N. York Acad. Med.,* 34:747, 1958.

JENSEN, H. P. (Germany) "Vitamin E for Spinal Disorders." *Munch Med. Woch.,* 102:1933, 1960.

JOHNSON, W. (N. Ireland) Letter to Editor. *Lancet,* 882:7129, 1960.

JOHNSON, W. F. *Science and Medicine of Exercise and Sport,* Harper Brothers, N.Y., 1961.

JOHNSTON, W. (Ireland) "Vitamin E for Athletes" (Letter to the Editor). *Lancet,* I:882, 1960.

JORDANO, D., AND GASPAR GOMEZ, C. (Spain) "Investigation into the Falling of Fighting Bulls during Bullfights." *Arch. Zootecnia,* 3:3, 1954.

JOSLIN, E. P. *J.A.M.A.,* 147:209, 1951; *J.A.M.A.,* 156:1584, 1954.

———— *Diabetes,* 1:490, Nov.–Dec., 1952.

———— "Diabetic Coma." *Penna. Med. J.,* 56:353, May, 1953.

———— *Diabetes,* 5:137, March–April, 1956.

JOSLIN, E. P., ROOT, H. F., WHITE, P., MARBLE, A., AND BANEY, C. C. *The Treatment of Diabetes Mellitus.* Lea & Febiger, Philadelphia, 10th ed., 1959.

Journal American Geriatric Society (Editorial) "Arteriosclerosis, the Concentration Camp Disease," 9:1100, 1961.

Journal American Medical Association "Vitamin E for 'Hot Flashes,'" 167:1806, 1958.

———— "Induration of Corpora Cavernosa," 168:1955, 1958.

———— "Arteriosclerotic Disease," 170:1753, 1959.

———— "Surgery for Aorto-Iliac Occlusive Disease," 961:179, 1962.

KAHULAS, B. A. (Australia) "A Myopathy Affecting a Marsupial, the Quokka, in Zoos, Reversed by Alpha Tocopherol." *Nature,* 191:402, 1961.

KALINICHENKO, T. J. (U.S.S.R.) "The Role of Vitamin E in Treating Spontaneous Abortions." *Soviet Med.,* 22:106, 1958.

KAMIMURA, M., TAKAHASHI, S., AND HENMI, I. (Japan) "Influence

of Vitamin E on the Low Oxygen Tension Tolerance of Mice."
Sapporo Med., 21:71, 1962.

KANNEL, W. B., DAWBER, T. R., KAGAN, A., REVOTSKIE, N., AND
STOKES, J., III (U.S.A.) "Factors of Risk in the Development
of Coronary Heart Disease—A Six-Year Follow-up of Experience." *Annals Internal Med.*, 33:55, 1961.

KAWAHARA, H. (Japan) "Alpha Tocopherol in Prophylaxis and
Treatment of Venous Thrombosis." *Surgery*, 46:768, 1959.

——— "Vitamin E in Prophylaxis and Treatment of Thromboem-
bolic Diseases." *Nagoya J. Med. Sci.*, 22:341, 1960.

KAY, J. H., HUTTON, S. B., WEISS, G. N., AND OCHSNER, A. (U.S.A.)
Surgery, 28:124, 1950.

KERN, H., MEISSNER, O., AND SPIES, R. (Vienna) "Treatment of
Arteriosclerotic Phenomena with Vitamins A and E." *Wien.
med. Woch.*, 108:178, 1958.

KERNER, I., AND GOLDBLOOM, R. B. (Canada) "Investigations of
Tocopherol Deficiency in Infancy and Childhood." *A.M.A. J.
Diseases Children*, 99:597, 1960.

KERRIDGE, D. F., MAZURKIE, S. J., AND VEREL, D. (England) "A
Clinical Trial of Prenylamin Lactate—A Long-Lasting
Coronary Dilator Drug." *C.M.A.J.*, 85:1352, 1961.

KHAN, N. G. (Pakistan) "Vitamin E and Liver and Heart Degeneration in Mice." *Pakistan J. of Sci. Indust. Res.*, 3:128, 1960.

KIMMIG, I. "Significance of Vitamins for the Skin." *Arch. klin. u.
exptl. Dermatol.*, 206:408, 1957.

KING, J. M., AND MAPLESDEN, D. C. (Canada) "Purkinje Fibre
Studies in Dystrophic Calves." *Can. Vet. J.*, 1:421, 1960.

KINSELLA, D., TROUP, W., PALMER, W. H., AND MCGREGOR, M.
(Canada) "The Paradox of 'Coronary Dilator' Drugs." *Can.
Med. Assoc. J.*, 86:222, 1962.

KIRK, J. E., AND CHIEFFI, M. (U.S.A.) "Tocopherol Administration
to Patients with Dupuytren's Contracture." *Proc. Soc. Exper.
Biol. & Med.*, 80:565, 1952.

KLOTZ AND DEBRAY (France) *Soc. Med. des Hospitaux*, 14:1, 1949.

KRAUS, H., AND RAAB, W. *Hypokinetic Disease*, C. C. Thomas,
Springfield, 1961.

KROFT, H. (Germany) "Animal Therapy with Emulsified Vitamin
A and E." *Tierärztliche Umschau*, 15:246, 1960.

KUNSTMANN, H. (Germany) *Medizinische*, 35:1195, 1955.

LAMBERT, N. H., AND PARKHILL, E (Ireland) "Preliminary Clinical
Report on the Treatment of Tumours in Cats and Dogs with
Vitamin E." *Vet. Record*, 71:359, 1959.

LEE, R. E., GOEBEL, D., AND FULTON, L. A. (U.S.A.) "Anatomical and Functional Change in the Peripheral Vascular System During Certain Induced Increases in Vascular Fragility." *Annals N.Y. Acad. Sci.*, 61:665, 1955.

LEVINE, H. J. AND WAGMAN, R. J. (U.S.A.) "Energetics of the Human Heart." *Amer. J. Cardiology*, 9:372, 1962.

LEVINE, S. A. (U.S.A.) *American Heart Journal*, 66:49–52, July, 1963.

LINDNER, E. (Czech.) "Therapeutic Value of Vitamin E in Disturbances of Spermatogenesis." *Intern. Z. Vitaminforsch.*, 29:33, 1958; *Ceskoslov. gynaekol.*, 22:359, 1957.

——— "Vitamin E Values in the Blood Serum." *J. of Palacky University* (Doctoral Thesis), Vol. 25, 1961.

LIVINGSTONE, P. D., AND JONES, C. (England) "Treatment of Intermittent Claudication with Vitamin E." *Lancet,* II:602, 1958.

LOEPER, J., AND MARTIN, P. "Hypotensive Action of x-tocopherylquinone." *Therapie,* 14:268, 1959; *Presse Med.,* 67:352, 1959.

LONDON, W. T., ROSENBERG, S. E., DRAPER, J. W., AND ALMY, T. P. (U.S.A.) "The Effect of Estrogens on Atherosclerosis." *Annals Internal Med.,* 63:55, 1961.

LUISE, R. (Italy) "Effect of Vitamin E on Liver Changes Caused by Barbiturates." *Acta Anaesthesiologica,* 9:249, 1958.

MACLEOD, J., AND GOLD, R. Z. (U.S.A.) "The Male Factor in Fertility and Infertility." *Fertility and Sterility,* 8:36, 1957.

MAGNIN, P., AND GABRIEL, H. "Favorable Effects of Vitamin and Cortisone Therapy in an Habitual Abortion Syndrome with Vascular Sclerosis of the Endometrium and Capillary Fragility." *Bull. Federation soc. gynecol. et obstet. langue franc.,* 11:300, 1959.

MASON, K. E., AND BERGEL, M. (U.S.A.) "Transfer of Leprosy to Rats and Hamsters Deficient in Vitamin E." *Fed. Proc.,* 14: 442, 1955.

MASTER, A. M. (U.S.A.) "Angina Pectoris—A Thirty-Year Progress Report." *J.A.M.A.,* 162:1542, 1956.

MATHIS, H. "Vitamins in Stomatology." *Deut. Zahn-, Mund- u. Kieferheilk,* 14, 1951.

McKINNEY, B. (Uganda) "Atherosclerosis in Wild Animals." *Lancet,* 2:281, 1962.

McCULLAGH, E. PERRY, AND LEWIS, L. A. (U.S.A.) "A Study of Diet, Blood Lipids and Vascular Disease in Trappist Monks." *New Eng. J. of Med.,* 263:569, 1960.

MEDINA, M. S. (Colombia) *Semana Med.,* 57:994, 1950.

MEHL, E. (U.S.A.) "The Use of Vitamin E by Athletes." *Kansas City Star* (Sporting Comments), Sept., 1962.

MERVYN, L., AND MORTON, R. A. (England) "Unsaponifiable Fraction of Lipid from Normal and Diseased Human Kidney." *Biochem. J.,* 72:106, 1959.

Metropolitan Life Insurance Company "The Increasing Chances for Survival" March, 1955.

——— "Health of the School-Age Population" *Statistical Bulletin,* August, 1961.

——— "Cohort Survival for Generations Since 1840" Jacobson, Paul H., Ph.D., F.A.P.H.A., 1963.

——— "Progress in Longevity Since 1850" *Statistical Bulletin,* July, 1963.

MEYER-WEGENER, H., AND LUZAK, E. (Germany) "Vitamin E for Blood Banks." *Klin. Woch.,* 39:754, 1961.

MINKOWSKI, A., SWIERCZEWSKI, E., CHANEZ-BEL, C., AND GIEBELIN, C. (France) "Tocopherol Deficiency in the Newborn; Transfer of Tocopherol to the Foetus Injected into the Mother During Labor." *Rev. espan. Pediat.,* 14 (81):339, 1958.

MIRSAGATOVA, R. S., AND SHEINERMAN, M. D. (U.S.S.R.) "Effect of Vitamin E on the Content of Chorionic Gonadotropin in the Urine of Pregnant Women Threatened with Abortion." *Referat. Zhur. Khim., Biol. Khim.* 1959, *Abstr.* No. 2887.

MOORE, T., AND SHARMAN, I. M. (England) "Prevention of the Injurious Effects of Excessive Cod Liver Oil by its Fortification with Vitamin E." *British J. Nutrition,* 15:297, 1961.

MORGAN, F. A. (U.S.A.) "Nutrition for the Aging." *The Gerontologist,* 2:77, 1962.

National Academy Science—National Research Council "Recommended Dietary Allowances." Publ. No. 589:25, 1958.

NELSON, G. (Canada) "Alpha Tocopherol for My Own Diabetes." *Summary,* 13:45, 1961.

Newsweek "Immune to Sperm" (Medicine), October 21, 1963.

NIELSEN, J. M., AND MARVIN, S. L. (U.S.A.) "Syndrome of Muscular Fasciculations and Atrophy." *Bull. Los Angeles Neurol. Soc.,* 23:51, 1958.

NIKOLOWSKI, W. (Germany) "Vitamin E in Dermatology and Related Fields." *Parfumerie und Kosmetik,* 8:1, 1956.

——— "Vitamin E and Skin Diseases." *Med. Klin.,* 55:415, 1960.

NIKOLOWSKI, W., AND ADAM, W. "On the Treatment of Oligo and Asthenospermia." *Proc. 2nd World Cong. on Fertility and Sterility,* Naples, Italy, May, 1956.

NISHIDA, T., AND KUMMEROW, F. A. (U.S.A.) "Effect of Dietary Fats and Vitamin E on Oxidative Denaturation of Low Density Serum Lipoproteins." *Proc. Soc. Exp. Biol. and Med.*, 109:1724, 1962.

NITOWSKY, H., CORNBLATH, M., AND GORDON, H. H. (U.S.A.) "Studies of Tocopherol Deficiency in Infants and Children." *A.M.A. J. Diseases Children*, 92:164, 1956.

NITOWSKY, H., AND GORDON, H. H. (U.S.A.) "A Role for Tocopherol in Human Nutrition." *J. Pediat.*, 55:315, 1959.

OCHSNER, A. (U.S.A.) *Postgrad. Med.*, 10:794, 1951.

OCHSNER, A., DEBAKEY, M. E., AND DECAMP, P. T. (U.S.A.) *J. Am. Med. Assoc.*, 144:831, 1950.

OCHSNER, A., KAY, J. H., DECAMP, P. T., HUTTON, S. B., AND BALLA, G. A. (U.S.A.) *Annals Surgery*, 131:652, 1950.

O'CONNOR, V. R. (England) *Summary*, 11:71, 1959.

O'CONNOR, V. R., AND HODGES, J. P. S. (England) *Summary*, 8:24, 1956.

PASSERI, M. (Italy) "Elimination of 5-Hydroxyindolacetic Acid in Human Urine." *Gior. Clin. Med.*, 42:589, 1961.

PETERFFY, P., KEREKES, S., AND FODOR, B. (Romania) "Vitamin E in the Pre-Operative Management of Goitre and Basedow's Disease." *Zent. Chir.*, 86:1541, 1961.

PHELPS, W. M. (U.S.A.) "Treatment of Dystonia Musculorum Deformans Progressiva." *Arch. Pediat.*, 78:169, 1961.

PIANA, C. (Italy) "Vitamin E and Repair of Wounds in Striped Muscle." *Acta Vitaminol.*, 6:69, 1952.

PICKERING, D. E., FISHER, D. A., PERLEY, A., BASSINGER, G. M., AND MOON, H. D. (U.S.A.) "Atherosclerosis in Monkeys." *Am. J. Dis. Child*, 102:42, 1961.

Pocket Books, Inc. *Royal Canadian Air Force Exercise Plans for Physical Fitness.*

POLLARD, J. W., HAMILTON, M. J., CHRISTENSEN, N. A., AND ACHOR, R. W. P. (U.S.A.) "Long Term Anticoagulant Therapy." *Circulation*, 25:311, 1962.

POLLER, L. (England) "Anticoagulants in Acute Myocardial Infarction." *Lancet* (letter), 2:983, 1961.

PROKOP, L. (Germany) "The Effect of Natural Vitamin E on Oxygen Consumption and Oxygen Debt." *Sportärztl. Prax.*, 1:19–23, 1960.

PROSPERI, P. (Italy) *Accad. Med. Fisica Florentina*, March 10, 1949.

RATCLIFFE, H. L., AND CRONIN, M. T. I. (U.S.A.) "Arteriosclerosis in Zoo Animals." *Circulation*, 18:41, 1958.

RICHARDS, D. W., BLAND, E. F., AND WHITE, P. D. (U.S.A.) "A 25-Year Follow-up Study of 200 Patients with Myocardial Infarction." *J. Chr. Diseases*, 4:415, 1956.

RICHTER, I. H., CLIFFTON, E. E., EPSTEIN, S., MUSACCHIO, F., NASSAR, A., FAVAZZA, A. G., AND KATABI, G. (U.S.A.) "Thrombolysin Therapy in Myocardial Infarction." *Amer. J. of Cardiology*, 9:82, 1962.

RODNAN, G. P., CHERNICK, S. S., AND SCHWARZ, K. (U.S.A.) "Reversal of Respiratory Decline in Necrotic Liver Degeneration by Intraportal Tocopherols." *J. Biol. Chem.*, 221:231, 1956.

RODRIGUEZ, G. F. A. (Peru) *An. fac. Farm. Bioquim*, Lima 7:42, 1956.

ROSE, IAN F. (U.S.A.) *Faith, Love and Seaweed*, Prentice-Hall, 1964.

ROSENKRANTZ, H., AND LAFERTE, R. O. (U.S.A.) "In Vitro Inhibition of Glycogenesis by D-Alpha Tocopherol." *Proc. Soc. Exp. Biol. and Med.*, 106:391, 1961.

ROVETTA, P., AND BONARETTI, T. (Italy) "Contribution to the Study of Post Infectious Degenerative Muscular Atrophy." *Neurone*, 7:53, 1959.

Royal Canadian Air Force Exercise Plans for Physical Fitness Pocket Books, Inc., New York, N.Y.

SAHA, H. (India) *J. Indian Med. Assoc.*, 23:428, 1954.

SALA, O., AND DE STEFANI, G. B. (Italy) "Use of Tocopherols in Experimental Acute Otitis." *J. Franc. Oto-rhino-laryng.*, 6:879, 1957.

SANCHEZ IBANEZ, J. M. (Spain) "Menopausal Symptoms Treated with Alpha Tocopherol." *Revista Espanola de Obstet. y Ginic.*, 10:247, 1951.

SARMENTO, V. M. "Treatment of Leprotic Amyotrophias with Vitamin E." *Hospital* (Rio de Janeiro), 57:319, 1960.

SAUTTER, H. (Germany) "Vitamins in the Therapy of Arteriosclerotic Chorioretinopathy." *Deut. med. Woch.*, 83:1514, 1958.

SBORDONE, G. (Italy) "The Retina and Avitaminosis E." *Annali di Ottalmologia e Clin. Oculistica*, 82:225, 1956.

SCAPELATO, L. "Infarto del Miocardio e Diabete Ed." *La Settimana Medica*, Firenze, 1951.

SCHMIDT, L. (England) "Seven Years' Clinical Experience in the Treatment of Rheumatic and Ischaemic Heart Disease by Vitamin E." *Summary*, 7:64, 1955.

——— "Coronary-artery Disease" (Letter to the Editor). *Lancet*, II:1341, 1955.

SCHWARZ, K. (U.S.A.) "A Possible Site of Action for Vitamin E in Intermediary Metabolism." *Am. J. Clinical Nutrition,* 9: Part 2:71, 1961.

SCRIMSHAW, N. S., BEHAR, M., ARROYAVE, G., VITERI, F., AND TEJADA, C. (Guatemala) "Characteristics of kwashiorkor [sindrome pluricarencial de la infancia]." *Federation Proc.,* 15:977, 1956.

SELISKO, O. (Germany) "Is Magnesium a Vitamin E Synergist?" *Naturwiss,* 48:556, 1961.

SHAFEI, A. Z. (Egypt) "Clinical Observation on the Lactogenic Effect of Vitamin A." *Alexandria Med. J.,* 5:194, 1959.

SHAPER, A. G., AND JONES, K. W. (Uganda) "Serum Cholesterol in Camel-Herding Nomads." *Lancet,* 2:1305, 1962.

——— *American Heart Journal,* 1962.

SHCHERBAKOVA, M. G. (U.S.S.R.) "Experimental Vitamin E Deficiency as a Model of Progressive Muscular Dystrophy In Man." *Arkhiv Patol,* 23:15, 1961.

SHINSKII, G. E., TELEGINA, K. A., SHEKHOVTSOVA, V. N. (U.S.S.R.) "Vitamin E in the Treatment of Lupus Erythematosus." *Vestn. Derm. Vener.,* 36:64, 1962.

SHUTE, E. V. *Can. M.A.J.,* 52:151, 1945.

——— (Canada) "A Study of Congenital Anomalies." Read at *First World Congress on Fertility and Sterility,* May, 1953.

——— *Alpha Tocopherol (Vitamin E) in Cardiovascular Disease.* Ryerson Press, 299 Queen St., West, Toronto, Ontario, Canada.

——— "Alpha Tocopherol in the General Field of Fertility and Reproduction." Read before *American Ass'n of Equine Practitioners,* December, 1956.

——— "The Prevention of Congenital Anomalies in the Human. Experiences with Alpha Tocopherol as a Prophylactic Measure." *J. Obstet. Gynaecol. Brit. Empire,* 64:390, 1957.

——— "Vitamin E in the Prophylaxis of Congenital Anomalies." *Fertility and Sterility,* 9:256, 1958.

——— "Dyspareunia After Age Forty and its Therapy in 52 Consecutive Unselected Cases." *Summary,* 11:45, 1959.

——— "Vitamin E in Chronic Poliomyelitis" (Letter to the Editor). *Can. Med. Assoc. J.,* 81:424, 1959.

——— "Should Spontaneous Abortion be Prevented? Vitamin E in its Management." *Can. Med. Assoc. J.,* 82:72, 1960.

——— *Summary,* 15:1, 1963.

SHUTE, E. V., VOGELSANG, A., SKELTON, F. R., AND SHUTE, W. E. *Surg. Gyn. and Obst.,* 86:1, 1948.

SHUTE, W. E. (Canada) *Urol. and Cut. Rev.,* 50:679, 1946.
———— "Acute Nephritis Treated with Alpha Tocopherol." *Summary,* 5:2, 1953.

SMITH, G., AND LAWSON, D. D. (Scotland) "Protective Effect of Inhalation of Oxygen at Two Atmospheres Absolute Pressure in Acute Coronary Arterial Occlusion." *Surg. Gyn. and Obst.,* 114:320, 1962.

SMITH, L. W., AND WORNE, H. E. (U.S.A.) "The Biochemistry of the Blood in Bronchial Asthma." *Antibiotic Med. & Clin. Therapy,* 4:515, 1957.

SOLER CANTO, J. "Vitamin E and Ulcers." *Rev. espan. enfermendad, aparato digest. y nutricion,* 18:745, 1959.

SPIRT, J. J., DAVIDENOKOWA, I. M., SEWRJUGINA, A. I. (U.S.S.R.) "Use of Vitamins A and E for Various Forms of Atherosclerosis." *Ges. Inn. Med.,* 17:431, 1962.

STARE, F. J. (U.S.A.) "Nutritional Challenges for Physicians." *J.A.M.A.,* 924:178, 1961.

STARE, F. J., VAN ITALLIE, T. B., McCANN, M. B., AND PORTMAN, O. W. (U.S.A.) "Nutritional Studies Relating to Serum Lipids and Atherosclerosis." *J. Am. Med. Assoc.,* 164:1920, 1957.

STERNBERG, J., AND PASCOE-DAWSON, E. (Canada) *Can. M.A.J.,* 80:266, 1959.

STORMONT, J. M., HIRSHBERG, E. A., AND DAVIDSON, C. S. (U.S.A.) "The Peroxide-erythrocyte Hemolysis Test. Experiences in Patients with Cirrhosis, Jaundice, and Polyneuritis." *Am. J. Clin. Nutrition,* 7:206, 1959.

STRITZLER, C. *Annals. N.Y. Acad. of Sciences,* 52:368, 1949.

STURM, W. (Germany) "The Value of Vitamin E in Internal Medicine and Its Related Fields." Read at *Congress for Spa and Physical Therapy* in Bad Elster, Germany, October, 1956.

SUARDI, L. (Italy) "Effect of Tocopherol on the Thyroid, Parathyroid, Pancreas and Gonads of Normal Rats." *Gazz. Intern. Med. e Chir.,* 63:2007, 1958.
———— "Relationship between Vitamins and Hormones." *Gazz. Intern. Med. e Chir.,* 63:2194, 1958.
———— "Urinary Excretion of 17-Ketosteroids After Intravenous Administration of Vitamin E." *Gazz. Intern. Med. e Chir.,* 63:2398, 1958.
———— "Urinary Excretion of Reduced Corticoids After Intravenous Administration of Vitamin E." *Gazz. Intern. Med. e Chir.,* 63:2630, 1958.
———— "Metabolic Modifications from Tocopherol Administration

in Normal Rats." *Gazz. Intern. Med. e Chir.*, 64:1394, 1959.

SUTTON, R. V. "Vitamin E in Habitual Abortion" (Letter to the Editor). *Brit. Med. J.*, 2:858, 1958.

SZASZ, A. "Vitamin E in the Treatment of Mongolian Idiocy. Influence on the Organism of Vitamin E Given from Birth Onward until Puberty." *Summary*, 11:49, 1959.

SZIRMAI, E. (Germany) "Improvement of Peripheral Circulation Through Vitamin E and the Objective Control of its Effect by Means of the Szirmai neo- or myographs and myotonometers." *Z. ges. inn. Med. u. ihre Grenzgebiete*, 13:479, 1958.

SZIRMAI, E., AND RUECKER, G. (Germany) "On Combined Vitamin A, B6 and E Therapy of Arteriosclerotic Peripheral Blood Circulation Disorders and its Angiomyographic Control." *Z. ges. inn. Med. u. ihre Grenzgebiete*, 15:222, 1960.

Taber's Cyclopedic Medical Dictionary (Taber, C. W.) F. A. Davis Co. (Ninth Edition, 1963).

TAYLOR, D. W. (Scotland) "Effects of Tocopherols, Methylene Blue and Glutathione on the Manifestations of Oxygen Poisoning in Vitamin E-Deficient Rats." *J. Physiol.*, 140:37, 1958.

TELFORD, I. R., WISWELL, O. B., SMITH, E. L. (U.S.A.) *Proc. Soc. Exp. Biol. and Med.*, 87:162, 1954.

TELFORD, I. R., WISWELL, O. B., SMITH, E. L., CLARK, R. T., JR., TOMASHEFSKI, J. F., AND CRISCUOLO, D. (U.S.A.) Air University School of Aviation Medicine, Project No. 21-1201, 0013, Report No. 4, May, 1954 (Randolph Field, Texas).

TOCCI, F. P., GREENLEAF, H. E., AND WORNE, H. E. (U.S.A.) "Preliminary Report of the Biochemical Alterations in Metabolism as Found in Peristatic Amentia." *Arch. Research*, 1:27, 1954.

TOLCKMITT, W. (Germany) "Relation between Nutrition and Vascular Disease from the Standpoint of Animal Experiments." *Medizinische*, 1959, 1288.

TOLGYES, S. (Canada) "Changes in Insulin Requirement in Patients Taking Alpha Tocopherol." *Summary*, 9:7, 1957.

———— "The Outlook for Life in Intermittent Claudication Patients Treated with Alpha Tocopherol." *Summary*, 11:9, 1959.

———— "Vitamin E in the Treatment of Congenital Heart Disease." *Summary*, 13:36, 1961.

TRAVIA, L. "Il Policlinico, Sez. Pratica," 57:1297, 1950.

TRUEX, R. C., NOLAN, F. G., TRUEX, R. C., JR., SCHNEIDER, H. P., AND PERLMUTTER, H. I. (U.S.A.) "Anatomy and Pathology of the Whale Heart with Special Reference to Coronary Circulation." *Anat. Rec.*, 141:325, 1961.

U.S. Public Health Service Report: "Chronic Diseases," 1962.

VACCARI, F. (Italy). *Cuore e Circulazione*, 35:164, 1951.

VANNAS, S., AND ORMA, H. "Treatment of Arteriosclerotic Chorioretinopathy." *Acta Ophthalmol.*, 36:601, 1958.

VAN VLIET, N. V. D. (Germany) "The Vitamin E Requirement of Mink." *Deut. Pelztierzuchter*, 30:27, 1956.

VOGELSANG, A. (Canada) "Ten years' Experience in Using Alpha-Tocopherol in Certain Cardiovascular Conditions." *3rd Cong. Intern. Vitamin E* (Venice, Italy), 1955.

WALKER, W. J. (U.S.A.) "Should the Patient with Mild Hypertension be Treated?" *Amer. Heart J.*, 63:28, 1960.

WALTHER, H. (Germany) "Therapy of Skin Diseases." *Deut. Med. J.*, 10:345, 1959.

——— "Oral administration of Vitamins A + D + E in Dermatology." *Therapie der Gegenwart*, 98:89, 1959.

WEDER, A., AND MISSURA, T. "Study on Medical Therapy of Various Forms of Deafness with a Vitamin A and E Combination." *Pract. Oto-Rhino-Laryngol.*, 21:55, 1959.

WEINSTEIN, I. M., MATHIES, J. C., KATZMAN, R., AND FORNEY, F. P. (U.S.A.) "Osmotic Resistance and Post-Transfusion Survival of Human Erythrocytes Stored in the Presence of x-tocopheryl disodiem phosphate." *Proc. Soc. Exptl. Biol. Med.*, 99:170, 1958.

WEINSTOCK, B. S. (U.S.A.) "Vitamin E for Painful Feet and Legs." *J. Am. Podiat. Assoc.*, 51:563, 1961.

WENIG, H., AND WESTPHAL, J. (Germany) "Treatment of Scleroderma in Newborn with Vitamin E." *Zentr. Gynakol.*, 80:1673, 1958.

WENNIG, F. (Austria) "Antioxidants and Liver Disease." *Wien. med. Wochschr.* 194, 1958.

WHITE, P. D. "Sudden Death" *The Atlantic Monthly*, Oct., 1963.

WHITMAN, E. J., AND McGOON, D. C. (U.S.A.) "Surgical Management of Aorto-Iliac Occlusive Vascular Disease." *J.A.M.A.* 923:179, 1962.

WILDER, R. M. (U.S.A.) "A Brief History of the Enrichment of Flour and Bread." *J.A.M.A.*, 162:1539, 1956.

WILLIAMS, H. T. G., AND MACBETH, R. A. L. (Canada) "A Controlled Study of the Use of x-tocopheryl in the Treatment of Intermittent Claudication." *Canadian Soc. for Clin. Invest.*, Jan. 20, 1960.

WISWELL, O. B. (U.S.A.) "Influence of Alpha Tocopherol on Dental Pulp of Rabbits Exposed to Heat, Cold and Hypoxia." *Anat. Record*, 130:448, 1958.

WISWELL, O. B. (U.S.A.) "Influence of Vitamin E and High and Low Thermal Environments on Weight and Body Temperature of the Rabbit." *Aerospace Medicine,* 33:685, 1962.

ZANARTU, J., AND HAMBLEN, E. C. "Oligospermia." *Ann. ostet. e ginecol.,* 73:938, 1951.

ZHIRNINA, N. V., AND STRONKOVSKIY, V. P. (U.S.S.R.) *Terapevti-chiestkiy Archiv,* 33:26, 1961.

ZIERLER, K. L., FOLK, B. P., EYZAGUIRRE, C., JARCHO, L. W. GROB, D., AND LILIENTHAL, J. L., JR. (U.S.A.) *Annals N.Y. Acad. Sci.,* 62:108, 1949.

ZWEIFACH, B. W. (U.S.A.) "Structure of the Capillary Wall." *Annals N.Y. Acad. of Sciences,* 61:670, 1955.

Page 13   migraine headaches

HERBERT BAILEY

is a veteran reporter who has worked for newspapers in North Carolina, Nashville and Chicago. During the past fifteen years, he has contributed significant medical articles to leading magazines, among them, *Pageant, Collier's, Better Homes and Gardens, Argosy, Science Digest.* He is credited with bringing national attention to the first large scale successful and practical use of atomic energy in medicine—a force which has saved or prolonged countless thousands of lives. Also Mr. Bailey wrote about the first clinical trials of hydrocortisone in the treatment of arthritis and other diseases. He first acquainted the American public with *ultra-sound,* as used in industry and medicine. (In Europe and elsewhere, ultra-sound was used for many years for treating various diseases before being accepted in America.) He directed the world's attention to one of our hitherto unhonored, yet one of our greatest medical heroes—Dr. Émil Grubbé, who first used X-ray in the treatment of cancer on January 29, 1896. As a result of the author's efforts, Dr. Grubbé was finally accorded the recognition due him by the medical profession.

Mr. Bailey is the author of several books on medical subjects, and founder of MAN'S FRONTIERS, an organization devoted to explorations of the unknown and the dissemination of information on generally suppressed subjects.

Page 88 - children
98 - arthritis